The Race of
Dementia

DEBRA TANN, Ed.D.

ISBN 978-1-64670-357-9 (Paperback)
ISBN 978-1-64670-358-6 (Hardcover)
ISBN 978-1-64670-359-3 (Digital)

Covenant Books, Inc.
11661 Hwy 707
Murrells Inlet, SC 29576
www.covenantbooks.com

Contents

Acknowledgments

First, I like to thank my Heavenly Father for allowing me to complete this book. The inspiration He poured into me allowed me to articulate on paper the thoughts that were on my mind and heart. When I think of my writings in this book and His Word, my meditative state takes me to Proverbs 16:24: "Pleasant words are as a honeycomb, sweet to the soul, and health to the bone."

I thank my husband, Chris, for giving me the platform to write. Your encouraging manner was reassuring by simply asking me regularly, "Did you write today?"

I thank my three sons for their unconditional love and quiet support. It is such a blessing to be your mom.

I thank my three daughters-in-law for loving my sons and making every effort to share their lives with Chris and me. Also, I just thank God for my one and only granddaughter. Hallelujah!

I thank my mom and dad for their prayers, understanding, and respecting my thought flows by allowing me to call you back when I was busy writing. You seem to think I can climb all mountains; so with Him, I do. Thanks!

I thank Emily for helping me navigate all of the nuances of the computer while writing the book.

In addition, for always holding me in such high esteem professionally, personally, and spiritually.

I thank all of my friends and family who love me, believe in me, and always support my goals. A robust thank you for the deep-rooted activism of all advocates on the battlefield fighting against Alzheimer's and related dementias. Thank you!

Finally and most notable, to each of the individuals who were so transparent with me as to share their heartfelt stories. They were stories of sadness, challenges, humor, triumph, and unmistaken love as a caregiver. Thank you for gracing me with your presence and allowing me to share your intimate story with others. My prayer for you…"And the peace of God, which passeth all understanding, shall keep your hearts and minds through Christ Jesus" (Philippians 4:7).

My Genesis

In the mid-1960s, when I was in the fourth grade,
I was on a live televised show entitled *Bozo Circus.*
Our class was on the show, and toward the end of
the show; I was selected to participate in a contest.
Unbeknownst to me, the contest consisted of me and
three other contestants jumping rope. As a little girl,
this was the neighborhood norm, and I was quite good
at jumping rope, especially Double Dutch. Yes, some
of you are smiling because you know how to jump too.
During this jump rope contest, I simply had to jump
longer than the other contestants to win the prize.
I was nervous, but I remember my classmates cheering for
me as I jumped my little heart out. I won the contest, and
the prize was a Suzy Homemaker Oven! Oh my goodness,
it was bigger than me and what a wonderful prize it was
for jumping rope.

I was especially excited to use my Suzy Homemaker
Oven over the weekend because we were traveling to
my grandmother's house to see my great-grandmother.
I recently learned my great-grandmother was residing with
my grandmother in Chicago. Hence, I planned to bake
her a cake from my very own oven to welcome her to the
city. She and I had a great relationship. She had a special
affinity for me as I often visited her in Mobile, Alabama

with my grandmother. Traveling from Chicago with my grandmother was always a treat for me. Actually, being in the company of my grandmother was such a delight with incredible interaction between us. As I prepared the cake with happy anticipation, my great-grandmother would be thrilled that I baked her a cake. Moreover, I thought my grandmother would be equally ecstatic of my baking prowess. She as did my great grandmother believed all women should know how to cook/bake, and it began as a little girl.

Needless to say, I could not wait to arrive! Once we drove up to my grandmother's home, I darted out of the car with my baked cake in hand. I immediately stormed into the door and greeted everyone.

As I approached my great-grandmother with utter joy and excitement to see her, she was unexcited. She did not greet me with her exuberant hug and kiss. She often referred to me by saying, "Come here, gal." I knew that was a true term of southern endearment coming from her, but I did not hear that beckoning either.

In fact, it appeared as though she did not know who I was and why I was standing before her with a cake that was still in its tiny baking pan. Why was she unresponsive? She looked at me as though I was a perfect stranger, and she displayed no emotion. I was confused beyond measure.

Years later, I wondered why my mother or my grandmother did not better prepare me for what I believed to be complete rejection. My little heart that I used to successfully jump rope was broken. I felt as though I should have been warned. In my despair, the only solace my mother and grandmother could provide were hugs. Instead, I wanted answers.

The intent of this book is to provide insight, truth, encouragement, resources, and perhaps some answers on the subject of dementia. What is more, this book will discuss specific racial groups that face alarming disparities at disproportionate rates as compared to others. We are now experiencing *The Race of Dementia*. How so? There is a literal race against time to find treatment and a cure. While simultaneously; it is wreaking havoc on millions of black and brown people.

What Is Dementia and Related Diseases Defined

There are many types of dementias, research reports ten primary types. Each of them has specific symptoms that are attached to various diseases. For simplicity, I will be discussing five areas: Alzheimer's disease, Vascular dementia, dementia with Lewy bodies (DLB), Frontotemporal dementia (FTD), and Parkinson's disease dementia.

Let us begin by operationally defining dementia. *It is not a disease!* However, it is the *symptoms* thereof. According to the Mayo Clinic (2019), *dementia* is a medical term used to describe a set of symptoms that are caused by changes in the brain due to disease or injury. Most dementia symptoms occur in people because healthy brain tissue deteriorates, causing a decline in memory and mental abilities.

Symptoms of dementia usually include but are not limited to memory lost, impaired thinking and reasoning, impaired language skills, and personality/behavioral changes.

The term dementia and Alzheimer's are often used interchangeably. While they are related, there are distinct differences between the two. Dementia is the umbrella term for an individual's changes in memory, thinking, or reasoning (the symptoms) caused by changes in the brain due to disease or injury. There are many possible causes of dementia, including Alzheimer's. Let's take a closer examination of the various dementias. These definitions are operationally defined by the Alzheimer's Association (Dementia Types, 2019).

Alzheimer's (ALZ) disease is the most common cause of dementia, accounting for 60 to 80 percent of all dementia cases. Alzheimer's is not a normal part of aging; it is a progressive brain disease. Two abnormal brain structures called plaques and tangles are the hallmarks of Alzheimer's disease and are thought to damage and kill nerve cells. Plaques are deposits of a protein fragment called beta-amyloid that builds up in the spaces between nerve cells. Tangles are twisted fibers of another protein called tau that builds up inside cells.

Vascular Dementia is a decline in thinking skills caused by conditions that block or reduce blood flow to the brain, depriving brain cells of vital oxygen and nutrients. These changes sometimes occur suddenly following strokes that block major brain blood vessels. It is widely considered the second most common cause of dementia after Alzheimer's disease.

Dementia with Lewy Bodies (DLB) is a type of progressive dementia associated with abnormal deposits found in deteriorating nerve cells. The presence of Lewy bodies in the brain can affect an individual's mobility, as well as the ability to think, reason, and remember. Early symptoms include hallucinations and problems with sleep. Men are more likely than women to be affected by DLB. In addition, there is a shuffling walk, stooped posture, and rapid eye movement (REM). This list is not exhaustive. Dementia with Lewy bodies is the second most common type of dementia.

Frontotemporal Dementia is a neurodegenerative disorder. That means it is caused by the loss of or damage to nerve cells (neurons) in the brain. Some people with frontotemporal dementia have dramatic changes in their personality and become socially inappropriate, impulsive, or emotionally indifferent, while others lose the ability to use language properly. Frontotemporal dementia tends to occur at a younger age, often beginning between the ages of 40 to 65. *Quick brain reminders: the human brain is divided into two hemispheres. Each hemisphere has four areas called lobes. Each lobe is responsible for different brain functions. Two of these lobes are the frontal and temporal. The frontal lobe, behind the forehead, is responsible for personality, problem solving, abstract thought, and movement. These are called "executive functions." The temporal lobe, regions behind the ears, is responsible for naming, language comprehension, perception, memory, and hearing.* (Italics denotes the thought of the author).

Parkinson's disease Dementia Parkinson's disease begins in a region that plays a key role in movement, leading to early symptoms that include tremors and shakiness, muscle stiffness, difficulty initiating movement, and a lack of facial expression. As brain changes caused by Parkinson's gradually spread, they often begin to affect mental functions (dementia symptoms) including memory, the ability to pay attention, make sound judgement, and plan the steps needed to complete a task.

An estimated 50 to 80 percent of those with Parkinson's eventually experience dementia as their disease progresses. Because Parkinson's disease and Parkinson's disease dementia damage and destroy brain cells, both disorders worsen over time. Their speed of progression can vary widely.

For discussion purpose, symptoms I have noted are not exhaustive. The list of dementia symptoms for each disease is a bit more extensive. My goal is to provide an overview. In addition to the above diseases that have dementia symptoms, I must include *Mild Cognitive Impairment* (Alzheimer's Association, 2019). MCI causes a slight but noticeable and measurable decline in cognitive abilities, including memory and thinking skills. MCI causes changes that are serious enough to be noticed by the individuals experiencing them or to other people. At this point, changes are not severe enough to interfere with independent function. A person with MCI is at an increased risk of developing Alzheimer's or one of the other diseases discussed earlier.

Facts and Figures

The most recent *Facts and Figures 2020*, according to the Alzheimer's Association.

- Alzheimer's disease is the sixth leading cause of death in the United States.
- More than sixteen million Americans provide unpaid care for people with Alzheimer's or other dementias.
- Caregivers provided an estimated 18.6 billion hours of care valued at over 244 billion dollars.
- One in three seniors die with Alzheimer's or another dementia. It kills more than breast cancer and prostate cancer combined.
- In 2020, Alzheimer's and other dementias will cost the nation 305 billion dollars. By 2050, these costs could rise as high as 1.1 trillion.
- One in 10 people age 65 and older (10%) have Alzheimer's dementia.
- 50% of primary care physicians believe the medical profession is *not* ready for the growing number of people with Alzheimer's or other dementias.

- Between 2000 and 2018, deaths from heart disease have *decreased* 7.8% while deaths from Alzheimer's have *increased* 146%.
- More than 5 million Americans are living with Alzheimer's. By 2050, this number is projected to rise to nearly 14 million.
- Most caregivers (66%) live with the person with dementia in the community.
- Only 16 percent of seniors receive regular cognitive assessments during routine health care checkups.
- Every sixty-five seconds, someone in the United States develops Alzheimer's.
- Older African Americans are about twice as likely to have Alzheimer's or other diseases with dementia as older whites. Hispanics are about one and one half times as likely to have a dementia related disease.
- Two out of three women in America have Alzheimer's.
- Alzheimer's disease is the only top ten cause of deaths in the United States that cannot be prevented, cured, or even slowed down.
- About one in three caregivers (30%) are age sixty-five or older.
- One out of three caregivers are daughters.
- One out of four caregivers are called "sandwich generation" caregivers which means they are not only caring for an aging parent but also children under age eighteen.

According to the Alzheimer's Association, as you understand dementia, your memory often changes as you grow older. Some people recognize changes in themselves before anyone else notices. In other cases, friends and family are the first to observe changes in memory, behavior, or abilities. It may be hard to know the difference between age-related changes and the first sign of dementia, but memory loss that disrupts daily life is not typical aging. Dementia is a slow decline in memory, thinking, and reasoning skills. The most common of dementia is Alzheimer's. Correctly pronounced it is Ahlz-high-merz.

It is a fatal disease that results in the loss of brain cells and functions. Dementias that are progressive and irreversible include Alzheimer's, Vascular, Lewy Body, Frontotemporal, and Mixed. It is also important to note, there are other medical conditions linked to dementia. These include Parkinson's, Huntington's, Creutzfeldt-Jakob, and even brain injuries.

Why the Name Alzheimer's and the Genetics of Dementia

History happens to be one of my favorite subjects. Hence, it was suggested to me to include the historical context of Alzheimer's disease.

Dr. Alois Alzheimer is the person recognized as the pioneer in this medical area. He was a German neuroscientist and psychiatrist. In 1901, Dr. Alzheimer had a patient by the name of Aguste Deter, a 51-year-old patient. Her symptoms mirrored dementia which included memory loss, aphasia, disorientation, confusion, hallucinations, and delusions. He spent extensive time with her and noted conversations and her symptoms in detail. He recalled her stating "I have lost myself" when she was unable to correctly write something. After her death 5 years later, Dr. Alzheimer performed an autopsy on her brain. He discovered post death, what medical doctors now recognize with patients with Alzheimer's, they have plaques, tangles, and cerebral atrophy. Distinctive conditions of an Alzheimer's patients. For many decades after Alzheimer's discovery, the medical and non-medical community thought the above symptoms were just typical of aging. It was not recognized as a disease until the 1970s based on neurological research. It was not until 1995 that we found Alzheimer's medical records documenting his care of Aguste D. and conversations with her, as well as a sample of her brain tissue. His notes gave us additional insight into Alzheimer's research and also allowed scientists to directly verify the brain changes he had described in his lecture. Dr. Alzheimer did not take it upon himself to name the disease after himself. His colleague and boss, Dr. Emil Kraepelin, who recruited Dr. Alzheimer to the Royal Psychiatric Clinic of the University of Munich, linked the name of Alzheimer's to Dr. Alois Alzheimer. (Heerma, 2017, p.1)

Due to the sudden early on medical and scientific interest and current increase in this medical field of study; the Alzheimer's Association was established in 1980. Since their inception, so many other organizations have also launched in search of a cure for Alzheimer's and related dementias.

Genetics of Dementia

An article on the genetics of dementia stated, we all know how children often take after their parents or grandparents. This is in part because some physical characteristics are passed down to us from our parents in the forms of about twenty thousand different genes.

Genes are the basic units of inheritance. They are made from DNA and are found within almost all the cells of our bodies, packaged in paired structures called chromosomes. In general, everyone has two copies of each gene, one inherited from each parent. Genes provide the instructions needed to build and maintain our bodies. While much of our DNA is the same for all of us, many genes will differ slightly from person to person. These differences partly account for the physical differences that make each of us unique. They also affect our chances of developing many common diseases. There are two types of differences that can occur in genes. The first are common genetic "variants." A variant is not a faulty or abnormal gene. Rather, some genes have multiple different forms (the variants), and people can have different forms.

Some are more or less common, but
for any of these genes there will be
a spread of variants throughout the
population. The role that each gene
variant plays in determining any of our
characteristics is generally quite small.
Most of our individual qualities reflect
the combined effects of many of these
variants acting together, as well as other
factors like our lifestyle or environment.
Inheritance of a characteristic that is
influenced by a genetic variant is not
simple; the inheritance follows a complex
pattern. (Alzheimer's Society, 2016,
p. 1–2)

In contrast, the second type of differences that can
occur in genes are called "mutations" which are rare.
The effect of a mutation tends to be greater and can
be harmful. A gene with a mutation is a faulty gene.
Sometimes a particular characteristic can be traced back
to a mutation in a single gene.

The inheritance of dementia can follow
either of these patterns. A few families
have a simple inheritance pattern due
to single-gene mutations. Many more
families have a complex inheritance
pattern due to multigene variants.
While inheriting dementia directly

through a single-gene mutation is rare, genes are thought to play some role in almost all cases of dementia. This is because the different genetic variants we all have affect our chance of developing the condition to some degree. Our genetic variants also play a role in determining how healthy we are in other ways, such as our cardiovascular health. This means that they indirectly raise or lower chances of developing dementia. Genes are very important in building and maintaining our bodies, but most of a person's physical characteristics and their chances of developing particular diseases also depend a lot on their environment and lifestyle. Whether or not we develop a disease can depend on whether we smoke, exercise, and have a healthy diet, as well as our genes and our age. This matters because people tend to think of the effects of genes as inevitable or completely fixed, but in most cases this is not true. (Alzheimer's Society, 2016, p. 1–2)

How well have you taken care of yourself? Begin today by ensuring cognitive assessments during your annual checkups as a part of your lifestyle.

Their Personal Stories and Takeaways

Hope's Story

Hope and I met over thirty years ago. When I had my eldest son, she called to see how I was doing. I just started crying, and my newborn baby was crying in the background. She asked me what was wrong, and I babbled through tears that my baby would not stop crying. I explained that I checked the diaper, fed the baby, made sure his clothes were comfortable, and I even rocked him but to no avail. She said, "Deb, that's a hungry cry!" I explained to Hope that the pediatrician said to feed my son only so much every so many hours. She said, "Feed that boy. He's hungry!" Two more sons later, I fed those baby boys as per Hope's wisdom.

Fast forward thirty years. We were planning a girl's trip in 2018. Hope had excuse after excuse regarding our travels. As she was talking, I was listening fervently because I have never known her to forfeit having fun. Week by week as I listened, she began to slowly open up about her forgetting her keys, getting lost, and misplacing her purse. As she laughed off these behaviors, they resonated with me because at this point, I had become quite knowledgeable about the various dementias. As I listened, I too began to release information from all of my research. I knew if I wanted her to continue confiding in me, I needed to be transparent to help her.

As I gained her confidence, she shared how she would look at the palms of her hands and the lines would be spiders, or she would see mice running along the floorboard, and when she would look back, the mice would be gone (hallucinations). She shared how she is always irritated, easily agitated, and volatile with her spouse. She also recognized like most people with the onset or early stages of one of the dementias that something was wrong. At times, Hope wanted to be isolated and struggled with depression. She often wept with me because it was such a scary time in her life and I would console her.

Going to the doctor was out of the question. She stated often, "They will not take my independence away by taking away my driver's license." She only discussed the specifics with me, but her adult children began noticing something was amiss.

She did not want to share her experiences with anyone including a doctor. After my sharing many similar experiences that I had read about, she continued to open up. I always prayed for her in the interim.

Eventually, I sent her a basic information packet about dementia. It took her a couple of weeks for her to call me, but she did, and she wept. I knew my next goal was to convince her to see a doctor. After many months of sharing my knowledge, encouraging, listening, and laughing, Hope finally made a doctor's appointment. She managed to go to one appointment but could not remember the follow-up appointments. She also shared how unsuccessful she was on the SLUMS assessment. This acronym stands for Saint Louis University Mental Status and serves as a tool to identify mild or early dementia.

As told by Hope, one of her funniest stories, during her first doctor's visit, she revealed as little as possible. She insisted on giving the neurologist a glowing report of how well she was doing but was unable to answer basic memory questions. As she prepared to leave the office without her purse and other belongings, the doctor called to her and said, "Aren't you forgetting something?" Initially, she looked perplexed, then laughed, and said, "Oops," and embarrassingly gathered all of her belongings.

Hope talks freely to me about her condition. She is seventy years young and looks every bit of fifty-five. Hope is fierce, funny, and a friend for life. It has now been eighteen months of encouraging Hope; she either asks me the same questions over and over, and I answer her as though it was the first time she asked. Or she tells me the same stories over and over; I just listen to them again. As of this writing, she is still trying to set another appointment as she has missed two. She either forgets or confuses the dates and times. She also asked me to speak with her spouse but gave me the wrong number. Eventually, I spoke with her spouse. He agreed with me that she needs a diagnosis, so we will know how to best serve her. I also asked him to accompany her to all doctor's appointments.

During my writing of this book, I have been trying to stay in close contact with Hope. She is progressing in her dementia symptoms but has yet to have a formal diagnosis. She called me the other day to share that she finally made it to her appointment after four months of missed appointments.

She chuckled and told me she was *not* completely forthright or honest with her answers to the doctor.

She is still threatened by having her driver's license taken away because of a diagnosis. Nor did she mention her hallucinations. I am confident the doctor was able to read between the lines. She disallowed her spouse in the office with her. He could not verify or deny what was going on in the home. Having that input is viable because Hope cannot paint an accurate picture. She joked and said he was not going to have her locked up.

I have noticed over the past several months she is far more repetitive, cannot keep her train of thought, and tells me how it is unlike me to not return her calls. Interestingly enough, I have returned all calls, sent text messages, and left voice messages on her phone. According to Hope, it is unlike me to not reach out to her. We find ourselves laughing about the good ole days more frequently.

In spite of it all, she never fails to ask about my spouse, sons, and granddaughter. Her sense of humor is alive and well. I am so glad to receive calls from her; God knows I try not to miss them. It is becoming increasingly harder to keep up with her due to her short-term memory lost. In the last couple of months, there have been circumstances in the family. Her doctor's appointments are the last thing on Hope's mind right now but never far from mine. Hence, she still does not have a formal diagnosis.

Takeaways

- Your loved one should never go to their appointments alone. Why? They will forget what the doctor tells them and what they should tell the doctor.
- If they are experiencing memory decline, they will not and cannot remember what to tell the doctor. They will generally answer their questions glowingly. The doctors need a loved one to paint an accurate picture of what is going on in the home.
- They are frustrated, angry, moody, and irritated. Often they do not know why, but the truth of the matter is that their mind is always racing with colliding thoughts. If you ask a question, and they say I do not know; believe them.
- Questions are very troublesome for your loved one, try to avoid them as much as possible. Soon you will find you are a great listener!
- Your loved one has difficulty with words. The right words are difficult at best to recall. They often process much later what is said if they have not already forgotten.

- They are afraid, which can lead to isolation. They sometimes prefer not to be around others because they are aware of their inadequacies and afraid they may say or do something incorrectly.
- Listen to your loved ones. Acquiesce all the time (unless it is detrimental to you or them). It will make your life so much easier to just agree.
- Your loved one will pay more attention to your demeanor/tone versus your words. They are processing words differently and with more difficulty. However, they can read body language well.
- Your love one will likely get turned around directionally. At the mall, grocery store, or even going to a familiar place they have gone time and time again.
- Their orientation becomes confused, and it becomes a quagmire for them. Apps are available to keep up with your loved one's whereabouts.
- Less is more! Try not to overload their overloaded mind.
- Your loved one may hallucinate. Listen and try not to act alarmed.
- If they are combative or aggressive, try very hard to not retaliate with the same behavior. If you do, it will likely become worse. Remember, their reasoning/rationalization ability is not the same anymore; it is impaired.
- Medication may help your loved one.

- Anytime there is a change in behavior and/or health, schedule an appointment with the doctor.
- Keep a journal of behaviors for recollection purposes. The doctor will need to know this information. So much is going to transpire with your loved one, you may not be able to recall it all.
- You must take extreme care of yourself mentally, physically, spiritually, financially, and emotionally.
- In several states, if a diagnosis is rendered, a driver's license is automatically taken away. In other states, the decision is left up to the doctor to determine when a license should be pulled even with a diagnosis.
- Pray

Faith's Story

Faith did not think twice when it came to bringing her loved one from the west to the east coast, so she and her family could provide care. Although she knew he was in the early stage of Alzheimer's, she assumed they could be his in-home caregivers with ease. The first couple of months seemingly went well, until the day Faith's loved one decided he could no longer walk. There was nothing wrong with his legs the day before. His mind told him he could not walk, so for many months, he did not walk. This was the catalyst that impacted the health of Faith's loved one. In addition to his refusal to walk, he called her belligerent names such as a bitch. Faith would call him out and ask him, "What did you just call me?" He would deny it each time, and she would remind him of what he said.

He told her with conviction, "Now, precious, I would never call you a bitch." Faith was undaunted even when he urinated on the floor, masturbated in front of her, and defecated on the floor. When Faith asked her loved one, "Why did you dodo on the floor?" He politely told her, "That isn't dodo." She insisted it was; so he commenced to eating his defecation to illustrate his point. He hallucinated regularly by seeing a demon on his bed. He asked Faith did she see it, and she said no. He also made howling sounds nightly. Faith's husband insisted he was howling on purpose. On the upside, often her loved one would do or say something that was simply hilarious. For example, he told Faith, "You are cold as an icebox" because she would not allow him to drink orange juice at will. He loved music. No matter what transpired just before the music, once it began, he was in the groove.

After months of working her demanding full-time job and caregiving; Faith realized they could no longer maintain the proper care at home. In spite of caregiver's assistance five days a week for four hours per day, it became overwhelming. He was physically too heavy for Faith and the caregiver to move in and out of bed and bathe. Unfortunately, a sore manifested on his hip due to a lack of movement. Moreover, he developed a sore on his foot because of the diabetes.

The choice of a nursing home was a painful but a necessary decision. Faith and her family visited the nursing facility practically on a daily basis. She stated sometimes she would walk into the facility and hear her loved one howling. She said she would smile and say, "That's my loved one." The night her loved one went to heaven, Faith dreamt she turned on the music, and her loved one was once again in the groove. When the music stopped playing, he took one final breath and died. She woke up from the dream, and a couple of hours later, the nursing home called to say her loved one had died.

This entire experience lasted less than a year from the time he was brought from the west coast to Faith's home. She now believes had he stayed in his home, his routine, his normalcy, perhaps he would have lived longer. I reminded her that she and her family displayed a noble act of kindness by caregiving for their loved one when no one else would.

Faith states, in spite of the colossal and often frustrating responsibility of caring for someone with Alzheimer's, she admits they did have some good laughs. He died thinking he was a billionaire. He said, "If you just get me out of this nursing home, we can go get the cash out of the bank."

Takeaways

- Try to live in their alternative world. What do I mean? As long as it is not detrimental to you or your loved one, buy into the billionaire story for example. What could it hurt?

- At some point, you must realize when you can no longer provide the care that is necessary for your loved one. Be honest with yourself. If you are a caregiver for your loved one, you have given unselfishly.
- When your loved one calls you a name other than your given name, try not to react. Remind yourself, it is not your loved one but the disease.
- If their mind says its dodo (defecation) that's what it is. If you challenge them with disagreement, they will try to show you. Just acquiesce, it is so much easier.
- Many times you will say, "My loved one is such a liar." Remember, they have little to no ability to cognate. In their mind, they are not lying. It is as real as real can get.
- Nursing homes are just one option. There are many other settings available to serve your loved one. My encouragement is to ensure the facility specializes in memory care.
- Asking your loved one a "why" question is often met with resistance. Most often they do not know why and surely cannot explain why. Their cognition is compromised.
- Your loved one's hallucinations are real to them. Faith's loved one was convinced a demon was on the bed. Refrain from being condescending or

trying to convince them otherwise. Try to divert their attention.

- Medication may help your loved one. Anytime there is a change in health and/or behaviors, schedule an appointment with the doctor.
- Keep a journal of behaviors for your recollection purposes. The doctor will need to know this information. So much is going to transpire with your loved one, you may not be able to recall it all.
- You must take extreme care of yourself: mentally, physically, spiritually, financially, and emotionally.
- Pray

Grace's Story

He was utterly difficult to live with! If you say up, he would say down, kind one minute and an absolute bully the next. He was always apologetic, but seemingly a short time later, he would return to his unkindness. Moreover, Grace's loved one had an uncanny ability to turn it on, the charm that is, and turn it off during opportune times. These are some of the classic signs and symptoms of dementia.

They are very nice around others such as in Grace's case, but one on one at home, they are quite challenging. Why is this? They can be a master of disguises. The last thing they want is for someone other than you (their loved one) to know what is going on with them. What is more, they muster and use all of their brainpower to be undetectable in the presence of family and friends. It takes all they have to conceal their impairments from family and friends. Afterward, the caregiver/loved one are then saddled with all of their ill behaviors.

Grace's loved one stated unequivocally how much he loved her. He went on to say he would never mistreat her in word or deed. However, Grace did not feel that love. In fact, he made her feel as though she was the enemy. She was regularly torn between loving her spouse and having utter disdain toward him. In her heart, she knew this was not her loved one, as her husband was a generous and a fun-loving sociable person. She did experience glimpses of positive experiences with her loved one from time to time. She pondered, "How can I sustain those fleeting moments of happiness?" She couldn't. Life was not as she once knew it with her loved one, and it was no going back.

Often, Grace would not know what would set her loved one off. He was unable to connect on an emotional level and displayed maximum apathy. The task of processing thought, articulating those thoughts and merely coming up with the words became increasingly difficult. Communication amongst them was confrontational. Short-term memory lost, mood swings, confusion, and getting turned around directionally were commonplace. Grace often felt helpless as she wanted to help but could not connect in such a manner that resulted in teamwork.

Her loved one's decision making, judgement calls, and personality changes proved to be difficult and adversely affected Grace's health. Grace struggled with living in the same home with her loved one. She contemplated establishing another residence separate of her loved one. She would take very long getaways, and he would plead for her return, assuring Grace that life with him would be better upon her return. She would return home, and sure enough as Grace stated, he would return to his old ways. The truth of the matter, the old ways never left.

As she so clearly articulates, "It is mindboggling to look at your loved one, and they look exactly the same, but their behaviors are the complete antithesis of what was once so familiar." Grace often tried reasoning, appealing, appeasing, and kindness but to no avail. Sometimes out of misunderstanding and frustration of the disease, she would give him a dose of his own medicine. This reaction created a battle between the two.

Grace stated her loved one became suspicious financially and felt as though people were ripping him off. In fact, according to Grace, he believed it was he who accumulated their wealth as though she did not contribute. What is more, he blamed her for any and everything that could possibly go wrong. Heartbreaking as it were, Grace remained in her home, watching the disease stricken her loved one.

Takeaways

- It is almost certain that arguing with your loved one will usually create more havoc in your home. Instead just agree, divert, distract, but most importantly reassure. This takes a lot of practice and patience!
- They will have difficulty explaining themselves and/or finding the right words to express themselves.
- They will forget! Where they are going, where they have placed items, what they are supposed to do on a given day, what they have said to you, or what you have said to them. Often times, they remember quite vividly the good ole days.
- Your loved one will experience confusion. This in and of itself can be frustrating for your loved one. This could trigger a mood change and a bout of unkindness.
- It is highly recommended that if you are experiencing Grace's disposition, you must take good care of yourself on a very regular basis. Get away as much as possible (mini vacations) and pamper yourself (regularly). You deserve it, and without it, you cannot take care of your loved one.
- Why does your loved one seem to take their frustrations out on you? You must tell yourself and often remind yourself, it is the disease, not your loved one! This takes daily training. It is a

struggle to not take things personally because it does and will hurt.

- Anytime there is a change in health and/or behaviors, schedule an appointment with the doctor.
- Keep a journal of behaviors for your recollection purposes. The doctor will need to know this information. So much will transpire with your loved one, you may not be able to recall it all.
- You must take extreme care of yourself: mentally, physically, spiritually, financially, and emotionally.
- Pray

Charity's Story

As all stories, Charity's story is both heartbreaking and compassionate. Her loved one was diagnosed with Parkinson's disease in his mid-forties. Based on his current symptoms, his condition has likely moved into Parkinson's dementia. Some of the changes have been the fact that he tires easily, suffers from dystonia, insomnia, constipation, mood swings, restlessness, and the inability to smell. He can no longer lift, nor walk or stand for any length of time. This is a complete contrast from the once healthy, vibrant, athlete he once was. While his disposition of being strong willed, and desirous of being in control is still intact. His erratic decision making, impulsiveness, and utter selfishness is rampant.

Post diagnosis, he enjoys pornography, fantasizes about having affairs, lies, uses profanity, paranoia, gullible, especially with predators on the phone or online. These are characteristics that her otherwise husband from years ago did not display. In fact, he is described by Charity as being a great provider, loving but disciplinarian father to their children, and capable of coping with adversity. He was also career-oriented and loved socializing.

Charity has spoken with his neurologist, did some reading on websites, and spoke with another spouse who is also coping with the disease. She misses going to church with her loved one, date nights, sleeping together, him being a God-fearing man, and his assistance with chores around the house. She is believing God will give them the desires of their heart, the things they planned prior to this diagnosis. She also wants him to realize it is God first then her. She wants them to experience great family time together before the disease takes its toll.

During our interview, I asked her direct questions, "What makes you angry?" She answered, "His lying, spending too much money, especially on things we do not need. Going on the internet sites that involve other women, making decisions without consulting me, admitting he is wrong." What also angers Charity is her loved one not doing things he is capable of doing; like preparing his own plate for dinner after she has prepared the food.

"What makes you happy?"

"When he is not on his cell phone. Also when he actually leaves the house, I feel free! When he does not ask the same questions repeatedly and/or his talking too much."

"What makes you sad?"

"When he is out of control and succumbs to his impulsiveness. This causes distance between us and makes me sad. His accusatory demeanor as he claims that I am not helping him to get better, when he does not listen, and uses his credit card insatiably. And finally, he always seems to have some rationale, no matter the circumstance."

"What frustrates you?"

"When he cannot move parts of his body such as his hands and feet. He is very heavy for me to maneuver. Also when he stutters, and I cannot understand him. I am also frustrated because we cannot travel as we planned years ago."

"What irritates you?"

"He is constantly on the cell phone! When he is on the toilet, watching television, driving, spending time with our grandchildren, and even when he is in a relax mode. The cell phone is my archrival."

Since Charity's family is rooted in Christianity, I wanted to delve into her Christian beliefs as it relates to the disease and the struggles in her home. I asked Charity, "What do you say to God?"

"I request daily strength, to understand my husband, and forgive him over and over." And she asked God to help her to forget all the things that make her feel as though she is inadequate. She went on to say that she believes her God will never leave or forsake her, and He is always in control. She also told God she wanted a servant's heart and to help her not to give up.

Charity stated she is unsure as to whether or not her husband intentionally tries to hurt her. She did express that they have the same problems/issues, and he does nothing to mitigate them. She has shared her feelings, thoughts, and hurts with him but to no avail. "I have so many running thoughts," she said. "Thoughts and questions such as, is there such a thing as midlife crisis for men? Back in the day," she said, "I did not have to compete with social media. The internet is a crisis in our relationship because it provides the temptation for my husband. Everything is so available, even women during his idle time."

The self-care that Charity utilizes includes listening to Christian radio, gardening, prayer, taking antidepressant and anxiety medication, and crying. "I am sharing my story because I know there are so many others living with Parkinson's dementia or perhaps one of the other dementias. I want them to know they are not alone," she said. Charity further stated, "This is a hard disease to cope with, and I want to know of others; so I can learn how they take care of themselves. We as caregivers must have a forgiving heart and not hate our loved ones even though they do things that hurt us." On the other hand, Charity believes it is important to let your loved one know when your feelings have been hurt. She does not believe one of the dementias should be a mechanism or channel to hurt others.

Charity foresees their life as a continued roller coaster ride. She said it is hard to handle someone like her husband, especially now that he has Parkinson's dementia. "I also feel as though I am sinking in quicksand," Charity said. "My life, our life, will never be the same. In my martial vows, I said in sickness and in health. This covenant unto the Lord remains true in my heart. I just hope he continually gives me the strength and sound mind to endure."

I asked Charity if she could write the ending of her story, "How would it end?"

"My husband and I would travel and serve as missionaries in third world countries. I envision us sharing the Word of God with those who do not know Him. We would also live a simple and peaceful life anchored in pure love. I cannot control what will happen tomorrow, nor the next day or even ten years from now. I am hoping that our Lord will find a cure for this dreadful disease. I just miss the person who I married."

When Charity stated her final sentence, I began picking up the pieces of my broken heart.

Takeaways

- A network to help you balance your home life.
- You must empower yourself with information.

- Utilize the internet and telephone to chat with others with similar experiences, search clinical trials, reach out to support systems such as the Alzheimer's Association that provide counselors 24–7.
- Join a support group. It is difficult for the average person to understand the difficulty of living with someone with one of the dementias. You need to be around likeminded people.
- Do not isolate yourself. Taking good care of yourself cannot be overstated. It is not unusual for a caregiver's health to deteriorate exponentially.
- You can attempt to let your loved one know how you feel but it may become more frustrating for you as you articulate your feelings. Why? Individuals with dementia often lose their ability to connect emotionally with others. They often become apathetic which means they have a lack of feeling, emotion, interest, or concern, even about something of importance.
- They are generally indifferent and will not be able to reassure you with words, hugs, or sensitivity. You must arrive at a place by which you understand this piece as it will help you intellectually understand your loved can not provide that emotional support anymore.
  Yes, it hurts as that is an important feature in any relationship. However, your loved one cannot give you what they don't have to give.

- Some Parkinson's medication causes one to be hypersexual, which is a compulsive sex drive.
- Research or consult with your doctor(s) about all medications and their side effects.
- Resources are readily available. You are not on an island alone. People really do care and want to help.
- Try not to live in a perpetual state of sadness. Learn how to differentiate between the disease and your loved one.
- You must take care of yourself and pray.

Bathsheba's Story

In the presence of Bathsheba, there is an air of confidence and competence. However, that is external. Her story speaks to coping with a loved one seemingly in the middle of their dementia stage with degrees of functionality but experiencing far more glaring symptoms of dementia year by year. While Bathsheba appears to have a handle on working with her loved one, she expresses the daily challenge of coping. She said it never lets up.

According to her, she has learned to be pliable. She acquiesces a lot, and she said her new vocabulary consist of "yes, I understand, I agree, you are right, okay, and a smile." According to Bathsheba, her life is so much easier when she conforms. I asked her, "Has it always been this way?"

She laughed heartily and said, "No way." She said she has developed this technique over the years and employ it regularly. She said she uses these words to avoid what she calls landmines and to try and keep harmony and peace in the home. I asked her if her techniques were affective, and she said more often than not.

Bathsheba stated her biggest struggle is her husband's inability to express empathy and his display of apathy. It appears most often as though he does not care about her and shows a lack of interest in her life, according to Bathsheba. He also does not connect with her on any emotional level. This utter lack of insensitivity has been a hurdle for Bathsheba that she continues to jump over it. She said she is very lonely. She went on to say, "Simple things like hand holding, looking at one another with that special look, holding and caressing one another are things of the past." Bathsheba said she thinks he thinks they have sex regularly. She chuckled and said she further believes he does not realize they only have sex once or twice a year because of his inability to keep up with time and experiences. Bathsheba stated based on her experience with the Virtual Dementia Tour, she is not surprised if sex is the least thing on the mind of someone with dementia. She stated she would enjoy being held by her husband and being told how much he loves her. She said she cannot recall the last time he uttered the words *I love you*.

While Bathsheba's loved one exhibits many symptoms of dementia, he still maintains a lot of his independence. He still dresses immaculately, irons his clothes, and cares for and about his personal hygiene. He was once a phenomenal cook, but now recipes are harder to recall, and his food does not taste the same. She said, "He will often proclaim, 'I did the same thing as usual.'" She said she chuckles to herself because if he did the same thing as usual, it would taste the same. He does a good job of camouflaging the disease while in the presence of others. Primarily because those social encounters are light, airy, and fleeting. Recently though, Bathsheba describes a couple of situations by which she is noticing his decline. She stated two different friends gently stated that her husband did not know who they were. They said he had a perplexing look of curiosity when they encountered him. He is also using words in the wrong context and/or forgetting words that for him were common place like Merry Christmas. During the holidays, he was trying to say Merry Christmas but had difficulty expressing that thought. He was stuck and said Merry three times, the word *Christmas* was not recalled. He purchases exorbitant amounts of food when grocery shopping. The other day, he came home with twenty-seven peaches for two people.

Last year was a bit intense for Bathsheba as her husband became paranoid. He wanted the blinds closed more, thought they needed an alarm system for the home, and floated the idea of a handgun for the home. Bathsheba went on to say, they have shared the same home for over two decades without an alarm or handgun. What was so upsetting for Bathsheba is that her husband never shared that he had a loaded gun at the head of their bed. In fact, she found it dusting underneath the bed. He responded to her by saying, "What's the problem?"

And "I told you about the gun." Bathsheba said she
was really upset as they never discussed gun ownership.
She left for a week to try and process this occurrence.
She went on to say, "Trying to communicate with
someone who is highly irrational is not a rational choice."
Bathsheba stated that it was becoming increasingly
difficult trying to help her husband connect the dots.

His driving is impaired to the point that Bathsheba
drives now for safety reasons. She stated the driving really
made her petrified because it was almost like he was there
but not there. He displayed a glazed look while driving,
tailgating, driving at excessive speeds, and constant lane
changes. Bathsheba thought all of this was a recipe for
disaster. She said sometimes when she picks up the keys to
drive, he gives her no flack, then other times it is a battle.
I asked her how does she deal with the battle. She said she
just opts out of going with him if he drives because her
safety is quintessential.

Her loved one's attention to dates, events, time,
and orientation are really declining. Bathsheba has come
up with several techniques to cope with these areas.
Fortunately her husband is still managing his phone.
Sometimes when he sends photos to others, they are
from years and years ago. She said his phone is a lifeline
for him. He keeps a lot of pertinent information on the
phone such as medications he takes, his bills are set up for
auto pay via his phone, he plays games, and he keeps up
with his photos.

Bathsheba shared that her husband did an awful
lot of things around the house. He now struggles to get

things done and probably would prefer to not do them. It is certainly not due to laziness according to Bathsheba but because it is difficult for him to remember how to do something. Hence, she said there are several things around the house that he has tried to repair that was either put on backward or not working the same. What Bathsheba decided to do was use the things just as he fixed them.

He is doing things now that makes no sense. Bathsheba said she has no doubt it makes all the sense in the world to him. In communication with others, he is leaving out critical information and/or being confused with information given to him. He often does this with Bathsheba, but she is noticing he is doing it with others too. Bathsheba said she gets frustrated because he does not listen. What makes matters worse, she cannot convey, connect with, or rationalize with him. He makes every effort to showcase to his family and friends he is just fine.

After his showcasing, he is so depleted because it has taken so much brainpower out of him. I can tell it is getting harder for him to cover up, and others are noticing some things are amiss. "Toward others, he is jovial," Bathsheba said, "but toward me, he is most often cold, minimal conversationalist if any, isolated to his space, and seemingly in another world." I asked her how does she cope. She said much prayer, a support system, hobbies, and getaways. Bathsheba also noted her support system is made up of individuals who are aware of her circumstances. However, she says many supporters are just kind people towards her but unaware of her circumstances. She attributes this to the favor of her Heavenly Father.

Over the years according to Bathsheba, they have found themselves split up at the airport, lost in parking lots because she jumped out of the car without even looking, turned around on a cruise ship, traveling eight hours in the same state because he forgot his identification, and they had to travel back home to retrieve, and ensuring he goes in the right direction when he exits a building because he gets turned around all the time. Bathsheba said these are simple things she never had to think twice about. She said she has also had to learn how to do so many things on her own such as the elementary operation of the GPS. While minute, this and so many other tasks were handled by her husband. Bathsheba said she never had to concern herself with many household and outside tasks but that is now a thing of the past. Bathsheba said some days are better than others, but every day symptoms persist. She said from time to time, she has weepy and/or sad days, but she processes with prayer, and within hours she is bouncing back. While it is an ongoing challenge, Bathsheba said she has to persevere for the both of them. She wanted to consider clinical trials but as of this writing, she may be receptive, but he is not.

Takeaways

- Bathsheba is able to distinguish the disease from her husband. This has to be constantly replayed in her mind. It jolts her into the frame of mind that her loved one is not purposely trying to under mind her. Bathsheba would remind herself in the heat of things, "My husband would not do…but the dementia would."
- It may appear as though she gives in to behaviors; when in fact, what she is really doing is achieving self-maintenance.
- She seems to be knowledgeable about what is going on with dementia. Bathsheba tries to take advantage of opportunities to educate herself by reading.
- She is honest with herself. Bathsheba is not trying to live in a world of denial; she knows it is going to become progressively worst.
- Bathsheba is strong because she needs to be. She works toward shielding and protecting herself.
- Trial and error has worked. She has taken advantage of developing techniques that work for her/them.
- She pays very close attention to details. She is able to recall his strengths and weaknesses in terms of his changing abilities.
- Bathsheba recognizes her new normal and adjusting as necessary.

- Despite the constant disruptions in the home, Bathsheba is committed to giving it her all.
- Bathsheba mentioned her loved one's inability recognizing people he has known for years. Memory is an issue with dementia, but dementia also affects the part of the brain that enables recognition of features and familiarity in human faces.
- It is not easy living, loving, and giving in an imbalanced relationship. Perhaps for Bathsheba, she is managing, because she recognizes and works within the blurred lines.
- She seems to be in tune with her vulnerabilities. Prayer seems to be monumental in her life.
- You must become the expert on recalling where you are directionally. They will most likely be unable to help if you are lost.

David and Michal's Story

Initially, when I asked David if I may come into his home and observe him and Michal, he said, "Yes, if you think you can handle it." I was anxious to interview this family as he was a male caregiver. Research points to the fact that women suffer more often than men from the disease. Needless to say, I was anxious to interview a male caregiver. Here is their story.

I spent some time with David's significant other, Michal, first. I have known Michal for some years and

I did know her pre-diagnosis. I found her to be sweet, soft-spoken, smart, a numbers wiz, and she loved to dance. Michal was diagnosed with dementia at the age of fifty-five. This is an early onset. According to the literature, dementia is increasing at an earlier age. During the last three years, I have only been in the presence of Michal once or twice a year. However, I had seen the progression with my own eyes. Fortunately, when I first noticed behaviors, I had already begun researching this subject. When she responded to me as though she did not know who I was, I was not put off. I knew what was going on. David had also shared her condition with close friends. If she did not know me three years ago, I knew she would not know me while visiting in her home to collect this information. It is not uncommon to see decline over three years. Decline is most times gradual but noticeable and inevitable.

I knew I wanted to spend time with Michal first if possible. While I wanted to spend time with her, it did not necessarily translate to her wanting to spend time with me. Often they can be elusive, but fortunately it worked out for me. I found her to exhibit some of the classic dementia symptoms. I am going to enumerate what I experienced then elaborate on each. She was reclusive, sometimes combative; she had extreme difficulty with word association. Michal had a healthy appetite. She was non-conversational unless one took the time to communicate with her. She was frustrated with her electronics, highly repetitious, and unaware of most surroundings. Michal was in her bedroom all day.

It was her haven. Shades were drawn, and the room was illuminated with her electronics.

The first day at her home in late afternoon, she was friendly and lucid. However, on midmorning the next day, she was a bit more combative. Based on my knowledge and experience, I was able to calm her down and reassure her. She told me she could not remember my name, and she did not, but that was okay as I did not expect her to. When I took her back down memory lane, we talked about the birth of her daughter. That exchange was very short but meaningful because I connected with her. She and I are the same age. I initially tried to take her back to her high school days, but that did not resonate. Quizzically, she asked, "What is high school?" Hence, I then selected the birth of her daughter.

This subject matter lifted her heart immensely; it was an apparent happy place for her. The disassociation with words proved to be a challenge for me, but I was up for it. I had to constantly think of ways to frame conversation. I noticed she drank a lot of sweet tea. I asked her if she likes water. She asked, "What is water?" A bottle of water was near me, and I held it up. She said she has water in her mouth; she was referring to the saliva. She went on to say she only drinks sweet tea. I was running a quick errand, and I asked her did she want some ice cream. She asked, "What is ice cream?" I asked Siri for an image, and I showed her the photos of ice cream. She smiled, and I knew I was on to something. Henceforth, I used images to facilitate conversation.

At her bedside and in her bed, she has the TV remote, laptop, and cell phone. The TV remote was often referred to as stupid as she stated it did not work. Stupid as well as a few selective profane words were often used by Michal. I am convinced the TV remote worked fine, but she could not remember its operation. I could not help her because TV remotes change from household to household, and I do not troubleshoot. However, I did determine the TV is on the Game Show network all day. Her laptop is utilized for photo recognition. She somehow associates photos with people she may know. Her cell phone is used for games. Michal has a plethora of games on her device, and she plays them ongoing. Her daughter sends her games, and they play together. I found her ability to play games on her phone striking. I watched her for hours, and it was entertaining for her.

Michal's appetite is good. She prepares her own plate, places it in the microwave, and returns back to her room to eat. Once her caregiver, David, tried to give her vegetables, and she retorted. She tried to scrape them off of her plate, but her caregiver was insistent. She soon retreated, but I checked her plate hours later, and she had not eaten those vegetables. She did repeat herself often. I was comfortable with this symptom. I just responded as though it was my first time hearing it. Michal told me she did not know where she was (location wise). That revelation conveyed to me her inability to process her surroundings. Even if her caregiver shared with her where they were, she could not cognitively wrap her mind around her physical whereabouts.

Michal referred to her inability to process as her "stupid mind." I asked her to not say that. I told her she has a brilliant mind, perhaps we connected because she smiled. I contend a smile is universal no matter the language or communication bearer.

Even though Michal complained often about her stupid dementia and the medicine being equally stupid and ineffective, I quickly redirected her conversation with encouraging words. Many times, we would just sit in the bed together. Perhaps it was soothing for Michal to be in the presence of another. I kept it simple by smiling, reassuring, and being in her presence. Michal, like most others suffering from dementia, pay close attention to body language versus words as their verbal ability is compromised.

David's story as it coincides with Michal as he is her caregiver. Their story is an eye-opener. David is my only male caregiver in the book. His perspective is riveting. David was a former military man and went on to fortify his career by retiring from the federal government after decades of service. I have known David for a long time. Our conversation flowed easily. As you begin to read this story, I must admit I did not always agree with David philosophically or with some of his approaches with dementia. However, significantly speaking, we did have common ground, Michal and her utmost care.

David said he noticed things were going awry when Michal could not pass the test to obtain the renewal of her driver's license and when she left for her standing hair appointment and found herself almost in another state. Obviously lost and probably confused. She was diagnosed at fifty-five, and three years later, car keys were taken away. On the job and in her management position, she struggled with people and their association with her. David was able to help obtain a social security medical retirement for her. She worked thirty years for the federal government, culminating with a stellar career featuring her full federal retirement.

When he described Michal's pre-diagnosis, it was with admiration. He stated she graduated with an undergraduate and graduate degree. She graduated at the top of her class and was quite skillful with numbers. They have always traveled extensively, and according to him, they will continue to do so.

David took Michal off of her medication for dementia a month before this interview. He stated it was not doing any good. He said they are now relying on doctors who are more interested in ensuring her vitamin levels are maintained, as well as her brain chemicals and hormones.

As I began the interview, I asked him, "When you think about Michal, what comes to your heart?"

He stated, "She is still Michal, just with issues." David went on to say nothing makes him angry about the disease because he believes dementia is a part of life. He said Michal will not return to her normal self. Now she simply needs triggers to jolt her short-term memory lost. He contended that if he continues to remind her of specifics (the trigger), Michal will soon remember.

He seemed to believe she has select memory. As a caregiver, David has attended a conference and reads on the subject of dementia. He considers himself to be the source of his own strength as he continues down the road of caregiving for Michal. He did remind me with a "but" God is in control.

A doctor did express the importance of exercise. This led me into the subject of routines. David does all the cooking. I asked about hygiene. He said although she bathes herself, she does not particularly care to get in the tub. She wears Depends after a couple of accidents. I asked him if he got angry when she soiled her clothing. He said he did not. I asked about her teeth brushing. He said he tells her to brush; if she does, great. If she does not, he says he only makes a big deal about it if there is halitosis. Otherwise, David said she gets her teeth cleaned quarterly because she is disinclined about teeth brushing. He said they go to the gym five times a week in the morning.

David said she does not like going, but he tells her they are not going home until she completes her workout. She does finally acquiesce. I was not surprised of her reluctance because generally speaking, trying to get your loved one to do something is met with resistance. A seasoned caregiver can, in most instances, coax a loved one into doing the things they want.

Their routine still encompasses a wide range of domestic and international travel. David stated that while she does not know where she is most times, he encourages her to take photos. He believes that will help Michal with recall information. I asked him about coping techniques for himself; he drew a blank. I extrapolated and asked about his frustration level while coping with the symptoms of dementia. He said he does not get frustrated because he will not allow people to frustrate him.

He did go on to say he does get pissed off when Michal embarrasses him in public places. I asked him how he handles it. He said he just leaves the restaurant, venue, or activity. Embarrassment is also displayed by Michal's loudness in public places, rudeness toward Caucasians for no apparent reason, and profanity.

What is striking to David is Michal never once used a profane word in the history of their relationship. As we began to further unpack the interview bag, I learned David does not like it when Michal continually "bucks the system" as he describes it. Let me explain, seemingly no matter what David says, Michal has something to say, and it is usually no and/or met with resistance. Obviously, David believes whatever he is suggesting, it is for her benefit.

When asked about the future and what will happen with him and Michal, he said either she will die before me, or I will die before her. He reminded me that one does not live forever. David said Michal will never go into a nursing/convalescent home. I pushed the envelope slightly by saying what if Michal's condition was not conducive to home care with him. He stated emphatically that she will never be "put away" under any circumstances. David does experience self-care quarterly for a week or two at a time. At said time, Michal's daughter, shares the responsibility of her care.

I asked some rapid fire questions. "What makes you happy?" David stated he is not happy or sad, just content.

"What irritates you?"

"Nothing," David said.

"What do you hope this book accomplishes?"

"I hope for nothing."

"What did you think about the Dan Gasby and B. Smith story?" I cannot disclose what David actually stated but he did say a man should never bring dirt into the home, respect the home. I wanted to know if David could write the ending of their story, "What would it say?"

He said, "The disease does not end our story. We will continue to do all the things we planned prior to the disease. The finality of our story would be the hopes that the disease does not progress."

Post-interview, David reached out with several afterthoughts. These final lines articulates the original words of David and my non-interpretability. He started his conversation by saying, "The disease does not destroy a person, only the mind can destroy a person. The disease and its definition were decided on by a man who never had the disease in life. The man who named the disease never realized that the mind is controlled by behavior. A person will never get their full memory back, but they can control the disease by taking control of their dementia, which is really a mind-set and can be controlled by the individual. Particularly if the people around them make them feel just as important today as they did prior to the diagnosis."

David continues with his thoughts by further stating, "In this world, people depend more on what a doctor says instead of researching and understanding their own medical condition. As far as I know, only God has the power to heal the sick or decide when they die. I don't understand why people think man knows more of their condition than God. Back in time, Blacks were not treated by the doctor and had better health than those folks who were treated by a doctor. Today, that is all they believe is what doctors tells them, and the doctor just reads a book and tell them what they think is wrong and recommend medication to build their hopes up instead of letting earthly things heal their illnesses. People fear the manmade name of a disease more than the disease itself which does not make sense to me but to each his own. I believe this is how a lot of people were brought up to believe in others, which is the easy way out. Doctors prescribe medication to patients for the profiteering of their medical practice. They experiment with elderly patients who are expecting full recovery results. This never happens, and that isn't living. It is considered living for others which gives them control over your life."

Takeaways

- Medication is not a cure all. The symptoms are still prevalent. The medication mitigates the symptoms. If your medicine does not work, try a different one. I suspect something will help. Often when a loved one is in their latter ages, eighty to ninety years, perhaps medication is not prescribed. Early onset fifty to seventy years may need a prescription and clinical trials. I trust you will make the best decision for your loved one regarding their medication therapy.

- I was encouraged by David as he did ask me about clinical trials. I was elated to provide information.
- Balancing vitamins, brain chemicals, and hormones are essential.
- Dementia does not have to be a part of life. Some people will have dementia and progress to one of the other diseases and many others will not. Yes, there are no absolutes, but brain health safeguards are important now whether you have dementia or not.
- Dementia *is* short-term memory lost in part. However, as time and the dementia progresses, there is no amount of triggering you can do.
- Caregiver, I implore you to stay connected to all available resources on a regular basis. You are not in this alone. Help is always available in so many forms, take full advantage.
- Exercise is very critical as is sunshine, human interaction, daily activities, healthy food, water, and encouragement.
- Reassurance is key as they live in an unsure world.

- Patience! You will lose it from time to time. Perhaps that means it is time for a caregiver break.
- Their absolute default is *no*. I am tickled by it because seemingly nothing is satisfying to them. I know you will do the best for your loved one, expect them to generally say *no*!
- Use your charm and love them into doing what you want. Remember the apathy piece is likely diminished and/or gone.
- You are seasoned or on your way to becoming a seasoned caregiver. However, you will not be a perfect caregiver.
- Know you. You must know what frustrates, irritates, angers, or embarrasses you. You should not ever be at a breaking point. If you go to the doctor's office and you are an emotional wreck, you have waited much too long for self-care.
- Take your highly recommended self-care opportunities regularly. What is regular? As often as you need it. You deserve it and so does your loved one.
- If you must place your loved one in a facility, I trust you have done all you can, and it has come to that decision. A memory care facility is highly recommended; they are unbelievably progressive.
- In my humble opinion and based on the research, scientists, researchers, medical doctors, memory care specialist, neurologist, health care providers,

and the like are working tirelessly to disrupt dementia.

- Our Heavenly Father does control the *quantity* of years on planet earth, but we control the *quality* of our life while on earth.
- As of this writing, unfortunately dementia will continue to progress exponentially. It is unyielding, and we must remain diligent for our loved ones to usurp dementia's authority.
- Pray

Rahab's Story

Rahab says she thought her husband "had lost his mind," and she was going to help him find it. Needless to say, Rahab had no idea what life was bringing to her front door. She said there were so many behaviors that she witnessed that she actually thought her marriage was on the brink. The behaviors were so unlike her husband; she wondered if she was going to put up with this new husband of hers. Rahab stated her husband became flippant, rude, selfish, intolerant, unpredictable, and short fused. Behaviors she had never experienced by him. He was also extremely forgetful, easily disoriented with direction, time, and place. He also struggled with simple math computation, sequencing, and keeping up with his personal artifacts. He would take off on trips with little to no notice and most often without her. When asked about his travels, he would provide answers as though he had no sense of accountability toward his wife, Rahab.

For several months, Rahab wondered who this new man was as it certainly was not the man she had grown to love decades earlier as her husband. She continued to watch and be utterly surprised as the initial months passed. It was as though it was a totally different personality embodied in the man she loved and cared for. In other words, Rahab said he looked just the same but acted totally different. While Rahab watched her husband's behavior over many months, she struggled with living with her husband as it was increasingly difficult. Rahab was on an emotional zip line. Initially feeling at her wits end, angry, frustrated, hurt, and wondering as she put it, "What the hell was going on?" She prayed regularly but cried more. She remembers vividly one morning, she was up praying and weeping.

Her husband came into the living room and sat across from her with some distance and asked her why she was crying. Rahab said she told him she was hurting. He just looked at her for a couple of seconds and soon said, "I am going back to bed." He never consoled her in any manner with words of encouragement nor caressing. At that moment, Rahab stated she knew this was medical as this was not her husband, the father of her children.

Rahab had the epiphany of medical concerns as opposed to him having a midlife crisis. She said it just popped into her mind…Alzheimer's. Rahab said she began reading, and of course, it was not Alzheimer's based on what she read. However, his behaviors were classic dementia or MCI symptoms. Hence, the journey began.

Rahab was struggling on two levels, coping with irregular behaviors by her husband and trying to convince him to see a doctor. Between managing those two fronts, Rahab stated that so many things had begun to flood her mind of behaviors by her husband that she had just shunned. She thought they were normal and/or never gave it a second thought. For example, she said they were heading to a concert, and her husband dropped her off to pick up the tickets while he was to park the car. Rahab said she grew weary because it was taking far too long to park the car, and the show was starting very soon.

When he finally walked in, she asked what took so long, and he said he got turned around parking the car. She told him, "No problem, glad you made it. Let's hurry to our seats." Forgetting and/or misplacing keys, we all do that. Forgetting dates, everybody mixes things up from time to time. Unbeknownst to Rahab, she did not know it was going to become progressively worst and fast.

Rahab vacillated between two worlds. The world of experiencing her husband for short periods of time and the world of her husband turning her world upside down. She stated on many days her husband would be present. She knew it, and that made her happy and hopeful for his return. However, hours later he would be dismissive, cool towards her, and noncommunicative. She maintained on what she now knows as self-care by recognizing when she saw behaviors that were the total antithesis of her husband; she knew dementia was present. This train of thought helped her survive. Rahab managed to convince her husband to go to the doctor, it took nine months. They went to the doctor's appointment together.

Rahab had a list of behaviors prepared to share with the doctor. After the first three descriptions of her husband's behaviors, the doctor stated he needed to see a neurologist. You must be wondering as was I what three behaviors did Rahab share.

She told the primary care doctor that her husband placed the milk in the cabinet; he was looking for crackers in the oven; and he had placed the Armor All for the tires under the bathroom sink. The doctor of Rahab's husband did share that her husband would not have come to the office if he did not know something was wrong. An appointment with a neurologist was scheduled immediately.

Rahab's loved one went through a battery of tests to determine what was going on. The process was to rule out what medical concern it was not. Tests included detailed blood tests, sleep apnea test, SLUMS test (thinking skills), neurological exam (reflexes, function of the nerves, balance and senses), imaging of the brain, psychological work up (evaluation of mood, depression), and input of loved ones observations. The battery of tests took approximately three months.

Rahab did not share much of what happened during the nine months leading up to the doctor's visit; I asked Rehab to share some of the things that occurred, and she did. As she shared her story, it was fixating. Rahab said her husband played lotto tickets; something she had never known him to do. He stopped going to church, and one day he was smoking a cigarette; something he had not done in over two decades. He began going to the night club with his friends when he traveled, getting drunk, and drinking almost nightly. He often created discord in the home by doing things and not sharing them with Rahab, especially around finances. According to Rahab, these were remote behaviors and unlike the husband she knew. She stated he once went out with his friend and stayed out all night, too intoxicated to drive home. Rahab said the next morning she went off! Her see-saw tittered from anger to tears regularly. She said he often talked about his childhood days, reminisced more times than not in the past. He became far too friendly with two different women whom he called his friends, one he met at a club and the other was a neighborhood friend that he grew up with. He reassured Rahab they were just friends, but Rahab said she wasn't having it. He did sever those two different relationships. Rahab said normally speaking, her husband would not have had such relationships and would also consider it to be an unacceptable practice.

Rahab went on to say he would lock himself out of his car countless times in a month, and a couple of times, he locked the keys in his running car. He would spend money insatiably. Rahab said he was never cheap to begin with, but he would be over the top with his spending.

Some days he would be kind, many days he would be unkind. He would go five days or so practically ignoring Rahab, and then on the sixth day, he seemingly reconnected as though nothing had transpired. He grew to have disdain when having to answer questions from Rahab. His answers were either short, curt, or met with a cutting demeanor of imposition. A common response would be, "Because I want to." From day to day, Rahab said she did not quite know what her day would entail living with him. Rahab said you constantly walked on eggshells. She prayed that the Lord would toughen her skin a bit so she would not wear her feelings on her sleeves. Anything that could go wrong, Rahab's husband blamed her. He seemed to be constantly mad with her and would not talk to her for days on end.

Rahab's husband mixed their toothbrushes, face towels, and when traveling, she said the interstate would be immediately to his left or right, and without question, he would strike out in the wrong direction. He notoriously forgot things daily, mix things up when grocery shopping, or think he actually been to a place when they had never been before and try to convince Rahab of it. When he routinely forgot to lock the doors at night, Rahab stated she would stay up just to double-check their safety without him knowing. He was cynical, moody, and defensive. His decision making was impaired as well. Rahab described a situation where her prayers once again sustained her. Their television needed repairs, and her husband stated he would handle it. Rahab said the repair person lived eighty miles away. She did ask why hire someone from such a distance, and her husband stated he was the closest who worked on our style television. While Rahab thought it was a bit odd because their television wasn't anything special, but she let it go.

Long story short, the repair person landed himself in jail on a couple of charges. Rahab and her husband had no television, and the repair person had been paid in advance. I know what you are thinking, as was I. Rahab ended up becoming a sleuth to ascertain their television. She called the repair person's wife a couple of times and built a rapport. She then was able to obtain her address, and they drove over unannounced and stated they were outside of the home and prepared to pick up their television. Rahab said she did not want to lose their money and the television. The wife was caught off guard, but Rahab said they retrieved their television and all the parts. Rahab immediately called a repair person in their city, and the television was repaired in two hours.

Rahab's face glowed when she talked about the times when her husband was present. During those times, she said she had glimmers of hope, but the harsh reality of the symptoms would soon reappear. She said she felt robbed of her husband. Her prayer life never ceased and continues to this day. During this growth period, she called the Alzheimer's 24–7 hotline a couple of times to ask specific questions for insight. She also visited a support group but said she never returned because she felt like they were all in the same boat. What is more, Rahab said she thought it was pointless to sit around and discuss/listen to one another's woes. Although she said each of them had similar experiences, she did not feel support groups were her avenue.

As I listened to Rahab's heart, it occurred to me why Rahab did not voluntarily fill in the blank space between the initial doctor's appointment and the nine months leading to a medical diagnosis. Rahab went on to say six of the nine months were profoundly tumultuous, and the other three months she was constantly recovering from her brokenness.

Rahab never left her husband as in separation or divorce. She said she often got away from the home to keep her head straight but returned to the instability of the home. Her husband is currently on medication. Rahab believes she could not live with her husband if he were not on medication.

Rahab says she does see the decline over the years, but the medication helps immensely. The instability has minimized, but it is still a challenge. I asked her, "Why didn't you just divorce him?"

She said, "While I had options, divorce was not one of them."

Takeaways

- It is very common to know something is wrong with your loved one, but you just cannot put your finger on it. Have tenacity and seek help because you are right by realizing something is wrong.
- They too often know when things are off-kilter.
- Initially, before a diagnosis, you will either hang in there or you will flee. Only you know how you

will respond to your loved one when placed in the situation.

- If you decide for whatever reason you cannot cope or you chose not to cope, make sure your loved one is in competent, capable, and compassionate hands.
- Answers like "because I want to" become scapegoat answers. It is common for them to have catchy/canned phrases they can insert because of their inability to articulate their thoughts with sentences and/or dialogued conversations.
- It is also commonplace to revert to childhood days or decades earlier. Remember, their short-term memory (who, what, when, where, and how) is depleting. Hence, their long-term memory is usually intact.
- They also have difficulty with parameters, judgement, appropriateness, and impulsiveness.
- You will have to develop a "tough skin" if you do not already have one. Please do not cry at everything they say and/or do. Yes, it hurts, but it must be placed in its proper perspective.
- Differentiate…you know your grandmother never used a profane word in her life, but now she cusses you out. What will you do? Quickly recognize your loved one from the disease.
- You may want to give in. Wait! Seek alternatives to help your loved one. Resources are plentiful, take advantage of them. If all else fails, you must then do what is best for your survival. You cannot

take care of someone if you are not together yourself. If you need to seek a therapist, do so because you deserve it.

- My Twitter feed lets me know resources are waiting for you. Reach out because someone will reach back.
- Medication does not make symptoms go away, nor does medication cure symptoms. Medication mitigates the symptoms.
- As Rahab realized early on, your loved one is not purposely trying to do you emotional harm. When we do or say something that hurts another, one typically stops short of hurting someone's feelings, select words carefully, or apologize. This is not typically the response from someone with one of the dementias.
- Your loved one may be a bit more outgoing, flirty/over friendly, or have a lack of filters. This is common due to their lack of judgement/boundaries as it becomes impaired.
- Try not to be surprised and or embarrassed if they do or say something unusual.
- Be as patient as possible and encourage your loved one, as well as yourself to get enough sleep.
- Pray

Sarai's Story

When I met Sarai, I was immediately attracted to her. She was witty, funny, down-to-earth, well-educated, and a very supportive Christian woman. My family and I visited a local church of which she was a member. She was responsible for the children's library at the church. My children were young, and naturally it was our propensity to encourage all genres of reading. Although we only visited the church a couple of times, I was more excited about seeing Sarai in the children's library where we always had great conversation.

After our short stint of visiting the church, Sarai and I maintained our budding friendship. Over a short period of time, we discussed our Christian ministries. She shared how she wanted to launch a Christian library for the general public, and my vision was opening a Christian school. Both of our ministries came to fruition, and we supported one another without hesitation. Sarai was considerably older than me, but that did not matter to me. I seemingly have always loved to be in the company of those who are older than me, and it holds true today. Both ministries did very well in our community.

Fast forward to the last couple of years, Sarai eventually had to give up her ministry primarily because of her maturing age and many of the characteristics that accompany it. Genesis Christian School took on the responsibility of her library as our campus had the space to accommodate her voluminous library. In fact, on our campus, her library required two full classrooms to house her life's work of Christian materials and books. As Genesis took on her library, she would assist with setting it up again according to the Dewey Decimal system. I forgot to share; she had a Master's degree in library science. Reestablishing the library at Genesis had to be done according to the Dewey Decimal system was a mandate. I actually felt good knowing she was no longer responsible for her massive works, and Genesis was a good home for it. She trusted me as she knew because of our extended friendship; I would take excellent care of the library.

It seemed as though shortly after we moved the library, Sarai began experiencing many health complications. She lived alone as her husband had passed away a couple of years earlier. Someone at her church was her guardian as I referred to them. They checked on her and did all the necessary things to ensure she was doing well, but she wasn't.

She was hoarding, not eating nutritionally, hallucinating, and calling the police department on a regular basis. She was convinced someone was burglarizing her home, and the police would not do anything about it. This led to her hospitalization and the eventual placement in a nursing home to rebuild her strength. She hated being there. I visited her once, and she said she researched the information and discovered the nursing home could not keep her against her will. Next thing I knew, she had checked herself out. It was hard keeping up with her, but I was thankful I had the contact information of her guardian. They really cared for Sarai and were amazingly patient with her.

She soon returned home, but it reached a dilapidated point. She mentioned to me on a visit to the home, a possum had gotten into the home and died. It was determined, based on the condition of her home, she could no longer stay in her residence. Her guardianship found a wonderful facility for Sarai as it became obvious, her mind was no longer intact. They could not have another call to the police department with her complaining of the burglars. At this point and over a very short span of time of perhaps two years, Sarai did not check herself out of the private facility, but when I visited, she would remind me she was only going to be there for a short while. I knew this was permanent for my friend as our friendship had a taken a different turn.

After church on most Sundays, I would visit Sarai. She did not know who I was, how we met, her life's work with the Christian library, Genesis, or anything about our relationship. On some visits, I would notice her having gone to the hair salon or her nails polished. I complimented her on how lovely she looked. She would say, "Oh, rats," and laugh. I would encourage her to play Bingo, and I shared that activity with her. Sometimes we would just sit in the chapel quietly.

I simply became, as she described me, the pretty Black lady who pushed her around in her wheelchair. I was fine with that role. Sarai is now in the presence of the Lord. The stunning compilation of her library is now in the competent hands of a church and receiving great usage.

Takeaways

- Patience is so needed with someone with Alzheimer's dementia or any of the other dementias.
- Intervention is a must when your loved one can no longer live on their own.
- If you have someone come into the home, prefer a nursing home, a private facility, or a family member taking care of your loved one, please have a plan. The cost varies from state to state, but financially it is staggering. Many individuals have great insurance and can stay in a private facility. Many cannot and a family member or spouse ends up taking care of their loved one. Nursing homes expect one to have little to no assets, or you pay the staggering amount. Many times your state will provide resources to defray some of the cost if your loved one is at home or in a facility. The cost of agencies fluctuates. Some are terribly expensive and others are not. Which begs the question, why the discrepancy? You must conduct the research and vet all agencies and certainly an individual who you are considering to be the caregiver of your loved one in their/your home.
- Cost is so subjective when it comes to care because what is expensive to me, may not be expensive to you. Do your research and have a plan.

- Sarai could not smell the possum decomposition as they often lose their sense of smell.
- She did give her guardians a difficult time along the way, as well as the staff at the facility. Thankfully, they were supportive in their care for her.
- Sometimes your loved one may experience expedient signs and changes in their dementia, while others may move moderately in their progression. This is hard to determine/gauge as it is highly individualized. Therefore, someone must be vigilant about the care of your loved one.
- Keep them engaged whether they are in a facility or at home. Do your best to encourage them to be active in at least one activity. Whatever the activity, *make sure* they win and you celebrate their winning!
- Again, as long as it is not detrimental to you or them, live in their world. Oh, rats, I was just the pretty Black girl that chauffeured Sarai in her wheelchair.

Warning Signs

In 2018, the Alzheimer's Association created a list of warning signs for Alzheimer's and other dementias to help identify problems early. Individuals may experience one or more of these signs in different degrees. If you or someone you care about is experiencing any of these signs, please see a doctor to find the cause. Early diagnosis gives you a chance to seek treatment and plan for your future. Italicized responses are generally a typical and normal age-related changes.

One of the most common signs, especially in the early stage, is forgetting recently learned information. Others include forgetting important dates or events, asking for the same information, and increasingly needing to rely on memory aids such as reminder notes, electronic devices, or family members for things they used to handle on their own.

What is a typical age-related change? *Sometimes forgetting names or appointments but remembering them later.*

Individuals with one of the dementias may experience changes in their ability to develop and follow a plan or work with numbers. They may have trouble following a familiar recipe or keeping track of monthly bills.

They may have difficulty concentrating and take much longer to do things than they did before.

What is a typical age-related change? *Making occasional errors balancing a checkbook.*

People living with one of the dementias often find it hard to complete daily tasks. Sometimes they may have trouble driving to a familiar distance or remembering the rules of a familiar game.

What is a typical age-related change? *Occasionally needing help to use the settings on a microwave or record a television show.*

They can also lose track of dates, seasons, and the passage of time. They may have trouble understanding something if it is not happening immediately. Sometimes they may forget where they are or how they got there.

What is a typical age-related change? *Getting confused about the day of the week but figuring it out later.*

Some people with dementia symptoms may have vision problems. They may have struggles reading, judging distance, and determining color or contrast, which may cause problems with driving.

What is a typical age related change? *Vision changes related to cataracts.*

They may have troubles following or joining a conversation. They may stop in the middle of a conversation and have no idea how to continue. They may also struggle with vocabulary, problems finding the right word, or call things by the wrong name. For example, they may call a watch a hand clock.

What is a typical age related change? *They know what they want to say, but they cannot find the words.*

A person with dementia may put things in unusual places. They may lose things and be unable to go back over their steps to find them. Sometimes they may accuse others of stealing. This may occur more frequently over time.

What is a typical age related change? *Misplacing things from time to time and retracing steps to find them.*

They may also experience changes in judgement or decision making. For example, they may use poor judgement when dealing with money or giving large amounts to telemarketers. They may also pay less attention to grooming or keeping themselves clean.

What is a typical age-related change? *Making a bad decision once in a while.*

Someone with one of the dementias may also start to remove themselves from hobbies, social activities, work projects, or sports. They may have trouble keeping up with a favorite team or hobby. They may also avoid being social because of the changes they have experienced.

What is a typical age related change? *Sometimes feeling weary of work, family, and social obligations.*

The mood and personalities of people living with dementia or dementia related diseases can change. They can become confused, suspicious, depressed, fearful, or anxious. They may be easily upset at home, at work, with friends, or in places where they are out of their comfort zone.

What is a typical age related change? *Developing very specific ways of doing things and becoming irritable when a routine is disrupted.*

Communication and Dementia

As the disease progresses, the Alzheimer's Association 2018 data states the communication skills of a person with Alzheimer's disease or another dementia will gradually decline. Eventually, he or she will have more difficulty expressing thoughts and emotions. Ultimately, the person will be unable to understand what is being communicated and lose the ability for verbal expression. The challenges associated with communication can lead to frustration. It can be helpful for you to understand what changes may occur over time so you can prepare and make adjustments. Anticipating these changes and knowing how to respond can help everyone more effectively.

Changes in the ability to communicate can vary and are based on the person and where he or she is in the diseases process. Problems you may expect to see at various stages of the disease include

- difficulty finding the right words
- using familiar words repeatedly
- describing familiar objects rather than calling them by name
- easily losing a train of thought
- difficulty organizing words logically

- reverting to speaking a native tongue
- speaking less often
- relying on gestures more than speaking

Tips for Communication in the Early Stages

- Try earnestly to not make assumptions about a person's ability to communicate.
- You are dissuaded from excluding the person from conversations with family and friends.
- Speak directly to the person if you want to know how they are doing.
- Take time to listen to how the person is feeling, what they are thinking about, and what they may need.
- Talk with the person about what he or she is still comfortable doing and what they may need help with.
- Explore which method of communication is most comfortable for the person. This could include e-mail, phone calls, or in person conversation.
- It is okay to laugh! Sometimes humor lightens the mood and makes communication easier.
- Be honest and frank about your feelings. Don't pull away. Your relationship and support are important to the person with dementia.

Tips for Communication in the Middle Stage

- Allow time for response so the person can think about what how they want to reply/say.
- Engage the person in one on one conversation in a quiet space with minimal distractions.
- Be patient and supportive. Offering comfort and reassurance can encourage the person to explain his or her thoughts.
- Maintain good eye contact. It shows you care about what they are saying.
- Avoid criticizing or correcting. Instead, listen and try to find the meaning in what is being said. Repeat what was said to clarify.
- Avoid arguing! If the person says something you don't agree with, let it be.
- Try hard to not overwhelm the person with lengthy requests that require complex thinking. Instead break down tasks with clear step-by-step instructions.
- Speak slowly and clearly.
- Ask one question at a time. Multiple questions can be overwhelming.
- Ask questions that require a yes or no answer. Example, would you like some coffee? Versus what kind of coffee do you want?
- Give visual clues. To help demonstrate the task, point or touch the item you want the individual to use or begin the task for the person.

- Written notes can be helpful when a spoken word seems confusing.

Tips for Communication in the Late Stages

- Treat the person with dignity and respect at all times but especially now. Avoid talking down to the person or as if he or she isn't there.
- Approach the person from the front and identify yourself.
- Encourage nonverbal communication. If you do not understand what is being said, ask them to point or gesture.
- Sometimes the emotions being expressed are more important than what is being said. Look for the feelings behind words or sounds. Example, you may say, "Do you feel good today?" They may answer yes, but their face is exhibiting discomfort.
- Use touch, sights, sounds, smells, and taste as a form of communication with the person.
- It is okay if you do not know what to say; your presence and support is most important.

Managing Caregiver Stress

Are you so overwhelmed by taking care of someone with a dementia-related disease that you have neglected yourself? Your own physical, mental, and emotional wellbeing? If you find yourself not taking care of your own needs, you may be putting your health at risk. In 2014, the Alzheimer's Association offered suggestions and resources to facilitate best practices. In addition, as a woman of faith, I believe in the Source. Hence, I will remind you of prayers of hope in a couple of pages.

Find time for yourself. Consider taking advantage of respite care so you can spend time doing something you enjoy. Respite care gives caregivers a temporary rest from caregiving, while your loved one continues to receive care in a safe environment.

Know what community resources are available and become an educated caregiver. Adult day programs, in-home assistance, companions, and meal delivery are just some of the services that can help you manage daily tasks. As the disease progresses, new caregiving skills may be necessary. The Alzheimer's Association offers programs to help you better understand and cope with common behavioral and personality changes that may occur.

Get help and find support. Seek the support of family, friends, coworkers, your faith community, and others who can relate to your situation. Online social networking communities and local support groups are good sources for finding comfort. If stress becomes overwhelming, seek professional help.

Take care of yourself and manage your level of stress. Try to eat healthy, exercise, and get plenty of rest. Making sure you are healthy can help you be a better caregiver.

Stress can cause physical problems such as blurred vision, stomach irritation, high blood pressure, irritability, lack of concentration, and change in appetite. Note your symptoms and discuss with your doctor. Try to find relaxation techniques that work for you.

Accept changes as they occur. People with Alzheimer's or any of the other dementias experience change over time and so do their needs. They may require care beyond what you can provide on your own. Becoming aware of community resources from home care services to residential care can make transition easier. So will the support and assistance of those around you.

Make legal and financial plans. Putting legal, financial, and safety plans in place after a diagnosis is extremely important so the person with the disease can participate. Having future plans can provide comfort to the entire family. Many documents, including advance directives, can be prepared without the help of an attorney. However, if you are unsure about how to complete legal documents or make financial plans, you may want to seek assistance from an attorney. An attorney specializing in elder law and/or a financial advisor who is familiar with elder or long term care planning is important.

You are doing your best and visit your doctor regularly. Know that the care you provide makes a difference, and that you are doing the best you can. You may feel guilty because you cannot do more, but individual care needs change as the disease progresses. You cannot promise how care will be delivered, but you can make sure that your loved one is well cared for and safe. Take time to get regular checkups and be aware of what your body is telling you. Ignoring symptoms can cause your physical and mental health to decline.

Ten Common Signs of Caregiver Stress

1. Denial about the disease and its effect on the person who has been diagnosed. *I know they will get better.*
2. Anger at the person diagnosed or frustrated because they cannot do the things the used to be able to do. *They know how to get dressed; they are just being stubborn.*
3. Social withdrawal from friends and activities that used to make them feel good. *I don't care about visiting or my activities anymore.*
4. Anxiety about the future and facing another day. *What happens when they need more care than I can provide?*
5. Depression that breaks your spirit and affects your ability to cope. *I just don't care anymore.*
6. Exhaustion that makes it nearly impossible to complete necessary daily tasks. *I am too tired for this.*
7. Sleeplessness caused by a never ending list of concerns. *What if they wonder out of the house or fall and gets hurt?*
8. Irritability that leads to moodiness and triggers negative responses and actions. *Leave me alone!*

9. Lack of concentration that makes it difficult to perform familiar tasks. *I was so busy. I forgot my appointment.*
10. Health problems that begin to take a mental and physical toll. *I can't remember the last time I felt good.*

Italics are possible responses as a caregiver.

Please pay attention to these aforementioned common signs provided by the Alzheimer's Association. They offer a glimpse into the stress a caregiver may experience.

Prayers of Hope

King James Version

"For I know the thoughts that I think toward you, saith the Lord, thoughts of peace, and not of evil, to give you an expected end" (Jeremiah 29:11).

"Peace I leave with you, my peace I give unto you: not as the world giveth, give I unto you. Let not your heart be troubled, neither let it be afraid" (John 14:27).

"But my God shall supply all your need according to his riches in glory by Christ Jesus" (Philippians 4:19).

"For God hath not given us the spirit of fear; but of power, and of love, and of a sound mind" (2 Timothy 1:7).

"Cast thy burden upon the Lord, and he shall sustain thee: he shall never suffer the righteous to be moved" (Psalm 55:22).

"Be careful for nothing: but in everything by prayer and supplication with thanksgiving let your requests be made known unto God" (Philippians 4:6).

"Come unto me, all ye that labour and are heavy laden, and I will give you rest. Take my yoke upon you, and learn of me: for I am meek and lowly in heart: and ye shall find rest unto your souls. For my yoke is easy, and my burden is light" (Matthew 11:28–30).

"And he arose, and rebuked the wind, and said unto the sea, Peace, be still. And the wind ceased, and there was a great calm" (Mark 4:39).

"He giveth power to the faint: and to them that have no might he increaseth strength" (Isaiah 40:29).

"Now the God of hope will fill you with all joy and peace in believing, that ye may abound in hope, through the power of the Holy Ghost" (Romans 15:13).

"Finally, my brethren, be strong in the Lord, and in the power of his might" (Ephesians 6:10).

Dealing with Anger

These are practical ways of helping you care for a person with memory loss and confusion. People with memory loss and confusion sometimes become agitated, angry, or violent. These behaviors can be very hard on caregivers and may even become dangerous. The following tips are designed to help you avoid and defuse angry outbursts (Richmond, 2007).

1. Remember that anger is a symptom. Try not to take angry outbursts personally. Remember that anger is often the result of loss of control or frustration. Look for early signs of frustration such as fidgeting. Try to distract the person before violent outbursts occur.

2. Respond calmly. Respond to anger and outbursts in a calm and direct manner. Make eye contact. Speak in clear, short, and easy to understand sentences. Approach the person slowly and from the front.

3. Look for physical causes. Check for pain, illness, or constipation. These can cause frustration and anger. Have a doctor check for problems with vision or hearing that may cause confusion. Some medications can cause

anxiety, hallucinations, or paranoia. Find out if medications may decrease symptoms.

4. Avoid confusion. Limit choices that cause confusion. Avoid situations with a lot of noise, activity, and people. Do the same things at the same time each day.

5. Plan for quiet times. Make sure your loved one is getting enough sleep. Alternate quiet times with other activities. Try listening to soft music or reading aloud.

6. Reduce stress. Notice if your loved one is acting lost, confused, or frightened. Calmly reassure them. Take a break if you are feeling angry or frustrated. Your loved one may react to your mood. Plan stressful activities such as bathing when they are relaxed. Allow plenty of time for all activities and give clear step-by-step directions. Try a daily walk to reduce stress. Provide soothing objects such as a stuffed animal.

7. Assess danger. Make sure the person cannot hurt his or herself. Try moving five steps back from the person to defuse the anger. Avoid holding or restraining the person. This may make the situation worse. If possible, avoid an upsetting situation or lead the person away from it. Try to distract the person with a favorite food or activity.

8. Keep yourself safe. If your loved one is violent, make sure you are safe. If necessary, stay out of reach or leave the room to avoid getting hurt. Call family or friends for help. If you feel unsafe

or threatened, call 911 or your local emergency number. *Make sure the dispatcher and law enforcement knows your loved one has dementia or one of the other related diseases.*

9. Evaluate episodes. After a violent episode, do not remind or blame the person. He or she may have forgotten what happened. Look at what cause the problem. See if there is any way to avoid the situation in the future. Remember that by responding calmly, you can sometimes help avoid outbursts.

10. Create a calm and safe home. Reduce clutter in the house. Provide good lighting to lessen confusion caused by shadows. Avoid changing living environments and caregivers other than yourself when possible. When a change or move is necessary, include familiar objects in the new home. Try to make changes gradually.

(Italics denotes the thought of the author)

African Americans and Alzheimer's Disease

The Silent Epidemic

While dated information, I personally think
the research you are about to read is overriding. It is
overriding research because it directly affects people that
mirror me, Black folks. I implore you to seek the medical
help that avails you to help you and your loved one.
I know as a person of color, we are generally embarrassed,
taught to keep things a secret, or have distrust with those
in the medical community. Racism and exploitative tactics
are certainly legitimate concerns and apprehensions,
but this disease is unrelenting. Therefore, we must take
advantage of early intervention and all the programs and
clinical trials that avail us.

I no longer want to be one of few at the table
of discussions, workshops, seminars, conferences,
and support groups when this disease is killing our
community. Invoking self-care alone for ourselves and
our loved one is not enough. Simply put, we cannot do
it alone. The disease is colossal, and we need to be an
involved community.

An emerging public health crisis among
African Americans (Blacks) emerged.

This report brought together for the first time an accumulating body of evidence about the scope and nature of Alzheimer's disease in African Americans. Each study is important on its own, but only when put together does the magnitude of the crisis become clear. Among the findings from research highlighted in this report: Alzheimer's disease is more prevalent among African Americans than among whites with estimates ranging from 14% to almost 100% higher; there is a greater familial risk of Alzheimer's in African Americans; and genetic and environmental factors may work differently to cause Alzheimer's disease in African Americans. Scientist are at a vital juncture in research. Advances in genetics and imaging, combined with our increased understanding of the mechanisms of Alzheimer's, provide immense opportunities to examine the disease in African Americans in ways that would not have been possible even five years ago. Without additional investment in Alzheimer's research targeted to all populations, but especially to African American, there is a danger that research will be stopped in its tracks. One of the most promising areas of research where additional funding is needed is the growing body of evidence that vascular disease may be key mechanisms in triggering the manifestation of Alzheimer's disease. Data from longitudinal studies suggest that high cholesterol and high blood pressure may be significant risk factors for Alzheimer's. The implications of these discoveries are enormous for African American, among whom vascular disease and its risk factors are disproportionately present. Effective therapies for primary and secondary prevention of vascular disease already exist, including cholesterol lowering drugs (statins) and antihypertensive medications. Now, observational studies indicate that these drugs may also protect against cognitive impairment and Alzheimer's disease. This is a line of scientific inquiry that must be pursued as aggressively as possible. Call to Action. This report laid out a plan of action that will require an unprecedented mobilization of public and private resources on three fronts: First, to accelerate the research to understand Alzheimer's in African Americans and to develop effective methods to manage and prevent disease. Second, to increase awareness of Alzheimer's among African Americans, to expand their participation in research and to get services and treatments to those who are affected by the disease. Third, to develop and expand affordable, culturally appropriate services, including assessment, diagnosis, and care. The research showed African Americans are hard hit by Alzheimer's disease. Age-specific prevalence of dementia has been found to be 14% to 100% higher in African Americans. While the rates vary among studies, three out of four report these higher prevalence rates. The cumulative risk of dementia among first degree relatives of African Americans who have Alzheimer's disease is 43.7%. For spouses who share environmental but not genetic backgrounds, the cumulative risk was 18.4% of these findings of familial risk, reported in January 2002, are based on family histories of the largest number of African American families ever studied for Alzheimer's disease. The number of African Americans entering age of risks is growing rapidly. Age is a key factor for Alzheimer's disease in all racial and ethnic groups. Over 10% of all persons over 65 and nearly half of those over 85 have Alzheimer's disease.

The number of African Americans age 65 and over will more than double by 2030, from 2.7 million in 1995 to 6.9 million by 2030. The number of African Americans age 85 and over is growing almost as rapidly, from 277,000 in 1995 to 638,000 in 2030 and will increase more than five-fold between 1995 and 2050, when it will reach 1.6 million. Genetic and environmental risk factors for Alzheimer's disease seem different in African Americans. Genetic risk factors seem different in African Americans and white Americans. APOE genotype alone does not explain the increased frequency of Alzheimer's disease in older African Americans. Data from large-scale longitudinal study indicate that persons with a history of either high blood pressure or high cholesterol levels are twice as likely to get Alzheimer's disease. Those with both risk factors are four times as likely to become demented. Sixty-five percent of African American Medicare beneficiaries have hypertension, compared to 51% of white Americans beneficiaries. They are also at higher risk of stroke (Data from the Current Medicare Beneficiary Survey). African Americans have a 60% higher risk of type 2 diabetes, a condition that contributes directly to vascular disease. African Americans have a higher rate of vascular dementia than white Americans. *APOE: There are three types of the APOE gene, called alleles: APOE2, E3, E4. Everyone has two copies of this gene and the combination determines your APOE genotype. The APOE is the principle cholesterol carrier in the brain. Screening and assessment tools and clinical trials are not designed to address the unique presentation of Alzheimer's disease in African Americans. Ethnic and cultural bias in current screening and assessment tools is well documented. As a result, African Americans who are evaluated have a much higher rate of false-positive results. *At the same time, there is substantial evidence of underreporting of dementia among African Americans.* African Americans tend to be diagnosed at a later stage of Alzheimer's disease, limiting the effectiveness of treatments that depend upon early intervention. African Americans are seriously underrepresented in current clinical trials of potential treatments for Alzheimer's disease, particularly in trials conducted by drug companies. This has occurred even though evidence of genetic differences and response to drugs varies significantly by race and ethnicity. A Plan of Action, as the largest private funder of Alzheimer's research, the Alzheimer's Association has invested nearly $120 million to find answers to the disease. We are providing research grants to encourage new African American investigators and research on African Americans at a number of institutions and are particularly proud of our early investment in some of the most important research described in this report, including the longitudinal study of African Americans and Nigerians at Indiana University. In 2002, a primary focus of the research funded by the Association will be vascular disease and dementia. We have also formed a Diversity Work Group of leading researchers working on Alzheimer's disease in diverse cultures to help us identify priorities for future research. The Association values its collaborations with the National Institute on Aging and we are gratified to see the results of our work together. As a result of a workshop on Race and Cultural Effects on Measurement of Cognition, which we

cosponsored the National Institute on
Aging launched an important initiative
that will address racial and cultural effects
on cognitive function and measurement.
While we accelerate the search for
answers, we have to do more to help and
support those who are dealing with the
disease right now. Alzheimer's disease is
underreported in African Americans, and
diagnosis often occurs at a much later
stage of the disease. That has huge
consequences. People are not getting the
help they need, and families struggle on
their own at great personal, emotional
and financial cost. Many miss the
opportunity for the treatments that now
exist, which are most effective in the early
stages of the disease. The Association is
working to improve care and support for
people with Alzheimer's Disease.
Through our chapters, we have stepped
up our outreach to African American
communities and are developing specific
tools for outreach, education, and
services. Through collaboration with the
Administration on Aging, we are
developing model programs that are
finding new ways to reach underserved
communities. (Alzheimer's Association,
2002, p. 1–7)

I found data as far back as 1998 (it is likely it goes back further) that stated Alzheimer's disease amongst Blacks continues to be at an accelerated pace. As you read these lines, the disease is attempting to disrupt our lives into the future. Bright Focus Foundation printed an article by James M. Ellison, MD MPH as recent as 2018. The article addressed the burden of Alzheimer's disease in our community and provided recommendations for the disparities with medical conditions, environmental factors, and hereditary factors.

> Finally, there are shortfalls to our body of research into Alzheimer's. All too often in the past, research has been conducted in populations that were easy and convenient to enroll in studies, and in many cases without regard to the need to explore differences in vulnerability, pathology, and treatment among diverse populations. As a result, Blacks are underrepresented in clinical trials of Alzheimer's medications, requiring us to assume or guess whether race and other differences in Alzheimer's treatment populations might have an impact on their treatment response and prognosis. (Ellison, 2017, p. 4)

African Americans are more likely to have vascular disease that includes problems with blood circulation;

they may also be at greater risk for developing Alzheimer's disease. Risk factors for vascular disease include diabetes, high blood pressure, and high cholesterol; these may also be risk factors for Alzheimer's and stroke-related dementia. We must all advocate both for more research on Alzheimer's and especially for specific investigations into the effects of Alzheimer's treatments on other at-risk populations.

Never before in history has opportunities been so plentiful in areas of medical technology, clinical evaluations, and new treatments. Hence, all must have access to the fruits thereof. Preventive care, early detection, special population research is undeniable (Ellison, 2017). And the church said Amen!

Hispanics and Alzheimer's

During my research, I discovered the Alzheimer's Association discussed Hispanics at length regarding Alzheimer's and other dementias. While Latinos Against Alzheimer's discussion centered on Latinos, I am culturally sensitive. Therefore, it is important that I share the distinct difference between Hispanics and Latinos. What is more, it will also explain why I did not consolidate my research for both groups.

Broadly speaking, according to research, even though, often the terms are used interchangeably. Hispanic is most referred to as persons that speak Spanish natively or have Spanish-speaking ancestry. Latino/Latina is more frequently used to refer generally to anyone of Latin American origin or ancestry, which includes Brazilians.

Hispanics are about one and one half times more likely to have Alzheimer's or one of the dementias as compared to Whites. Although Whites make up the great majority of the more than five million people with Alzheimer's and other dementias, Hispanics are at a higher risk for developing the disease. Why is this?

There are no known genetic factors that can explain the greater prevalence of Alzheimer's and other dementias in Hispanics than in their White counterparts. On the other hand, conditions such as high blood pressure and diabetes, which are known risk factors for Alzheimer's and other dementias in all groups, they are more common with Hispanics.

What is more, socioeconomic factors such as having a low level of education and income are also associated with greater risk for Alzheimer's and other dementias in all groups. Data from a federal survey of older Americans shows Hispanics are disproportionately represented among socioeconomically disadvantaged people in this country.

> Reports show these health and
> socioeconomic factors probably
> contribute to the greater prevalence
> of Alzheimer's and other dementias in
> the Hispanic communities. For clarity
> purposes socioeconomic disparities,
> such as the aforementioned areas,
> speaks to reduced access to health care
> and thereby, reducing opportunities to
> avoid or manage high blood pressure
> and diabetes which increase the risk of
> Alzheimer's. Research illustrates that
> Hispanics recognize the importance of
> a diagnosis but lag time between this
> recognition and a medical evaluation
> is worth noting. This delay means
> one is not receiving, at its earliest
> stage of the disease, necessary medical
> attention and treatments when it is

more likely to be effective. This is recognized as underdiagnoses and or possibly underrepresented. (Alzheimer's Association, 2010, p.1-3)

It is my sincerest desire that Hispanics strive to not be a part of the underdiagnosed population. The Alzheimer's Association has a designated link that has translated their information into Spanish.

Latinos/Latinas and Alzheimer's

The lack of knowledge of Alzheimer's is particularly problematic for older Latino adults given the disproportionate impact of dementia on this population (National Hispanic Council on Aging, 2015). In a 2013 study conducted by the National Hispanic Council on Aging found Latinos have several misconceptions when it comes to Alzheimer's. Healthcare providers reported that Latino older adults knew little about Alzheimer's disease.

According to the study, older adults stated that some people get Alzheimer's because they think too much, are stressed, or have personality disorders (National Hispanic Council on Aging, 2013). Further, missed diagnoses of Alzheimer's are more common among older Latinos than among older non-Latino Whites, resulting in families struggling with symptoms of Alzheimer's in the shadows without access to proper medical treatment (Fitten & Ortiz, 2001).

Latinos with Alzheimer's often experience a longer delay between recognizing signs and symptoms and receiving a diagnosis. This is a disturbing trend as research suggests that symptoms of Alzheimer's appear almost seven years earlier in Latinos than in nonwhites (Latinos & Alzheimer's Disease: New Numbers Behind the Crisis, 2019).

Arturo, a caregiver for his mother with dementia, stated that there had been situations when we walked into the house, and the gas has been on for some time and her not realizing because over time, she's also lost her sense of smell… it was points like that where we realized, "Okay, she needs 24–7 care." (Latinos & Alzheimer's Disease: New Numbers Behind the Crisis, 2019, p. 10)

Those intimate words from Arturo articulate the heartbreak and destruction of dementia and other associated diseases. Dementia can be prolonging no doubt, and one of the classic symptoms is the declining sense of smell. However, researchers say there is a silver lining with this inability; it could lead to early diagnosis. Looking ahead,

The United States Census Bureau, projects that the Latino population will double from approximately 49 million in 2009 to 106 million people by the year 2050. In fact, 2044, more than half of all Americans are projected to belong to a minority group. The growth of the Latino community will have tremendous implications for our nation's health, education, and workforce sectors. It is essential that our nation's

policymakers and community leaders
better understand these consequences
to adequately address the public health
needs of an increasingly multicultural
society. (Latinos & Alzheimer's Disease:
New Numbers Behind the Crisis,
2019, p. 9)

Women at Risk

As in Blacks, Hispanics, and Latinos, women are also in the higher risk of one of the dementias. As in minority races and the general population, there is an overall race for a cure as women too are adversely affected. We have so much to accomplish in terms of research and seemingly so little time to eradicate dementia and other related dementias.

Alzheimer's disease is fatal. It is the only cause of death among the top 10 in America that cannot be prevented, cured, or even slowed. Of the more than 5 million Americans of all ages living with Alzheimer's dementia, the majority are women. Almost two out of three Americans with Alzheimer's are women. Of the 5.6 million people age 65 and older with Alzheimer's in the United States, 3.5 million are women. As real a concern as breast cancer is to women's health, women in their 60s are about twice as likely to develop Alzheimer's during the rest of their lives as they are to develop breast cancer. There are a number of potential

biological and social reasons why more
women than men have Alzheimer's or
other dementias. The prevailing view has
been that this discrepancy is due to the
fact that women live longer than men
on average and older age is the greatest
risk factor for Alzheimer's. Researchers
are now questioning whether the risk of
Alzheimer's could actually be higher for
women at any given age due to biological
or genetic variations or differences in life
experiences. (Alzheimer's Association,
2019, p. 1-5)

In 2018 in Chicago, the Alzheimer's Association
International Conference presented extensive research on
why women develop Alzheimer's or other dementias more
so than men. The studies were most interesting as one
presenter drew a correlation between dementia risk for the
first time to reproductive factors such as the number of
pregnancies or miscarriages a woman has experienced and
rethinking the impact of hormone therapy on cognition
was among the many topics of sex/gender-based research.
Alzheimer's Chief Science Officer, Maria Carrillo, PhD
was quoted as saying, "More research is needed in this
area, because having a better understanding of sex-specific
risk factors across the lifespan may help us discover
and eventually apply specific prevention strategies for
different populations of people with Alzheimer's and
other dementias." For further reading, please refer to

the Alzheimer's Association website and the findings/
discussion discovered at the 2018 AAIC Conference.

According to Maria Shriver, she believes her mission
is to wipe our Alzheimer's. She stated further on her
website that the disease is destroying millions of lives of
patients and caregivers. In 2003, her father was diagnosed
with Alzheimer's and post diagnoses; she has not stop
fighting for a cure. Shriver stated that two out of three
brains that develop Alzheimer's disease belong to women.
She wants to know why that is so. She launched the
Women's Alzheimer's Movement, which seeks to raise the
stakes for women based research. Visit her website for
further edification (thewomensalzheimersmovement.org).

Award-winning author Marita Golden wrote a book
entitled *The Wide Circumference of Love*. This book
takes you on a journey of a Black family coping with
Alzheimer's. In addition to many of her written works,
she also wrote a piece on a controversial issue that brewed
in February 2019. The subject matter involved B. Smith
who was then suffering from Alzheimer's. Golden wrote,

> Marriage, too, inevitably has been
> impacted, as more and more caregivers
> decide that they have a right to emotional
> wellbeing. B. Smith is no longer the wife
> of Dan Gasby, not in any way that we
> define a wife as an emotional partner
> who is cognizant of her partner's needs,
> desires, and can co-create a relationship.
> (The Root, 2019, p. 1-6)

Prior to this dreadful disease, B. Smith was a renowned model, author, businesswoman, and restaurateur. She was diagnosed with Alzheimer's in 2013. Her husband has spoken out often to various media outlets over the years sharing their story. They wrote a book together entitled *Before I forget Love: Hope, Help, and Acceptance in Our Fight Against Alzheimer's*. However, in February 2019, he went public with his now female significant other and how she has moved into their home to serve as a caregiver for B. Smith. Social media went wild! Many people had their personal spin on B. Smith's husband, Dan, and his many personal appearances on national television defending his position. Perhaps the concern was the fact that he brought his girlfriend into their home. Many felt Mr. Gasby displayed a lack of disrespect and certainly a lack of discretion.

Golden further stated, Dan Gasby is providing an alternative model, and he is willing to be the point person for a long conversation about the lives and needs of America's caregivers, who comprise an unpaid, silent, unrecognized army keeping families together (The Root, 2019).

Dan Gasby stated on all occasions that B. Smith told him to "go on with his life, to be happy." Hence, Marita Golden's written piece requested each of us to individually search our hearts and find compassion for caregivers. Personally speaking, I hope you never have to walk in the shoes of a caregiver facing the symptoms of dementia or other related diseases (B. Smith died February 2020).

Determining When to See the Physician and a Diagnosis

When you or a loved one have memory problems or other dementia symptoms, you may recognize such changes. Remember, as one ages, you will forget things as this is a natural progression of aging. The difference is when you forget and cannot back track your steps to retrieve and/or recall your items/information. For instance, you have gone to a particular store in the community for years. All of a sudden, you are driving to that same store, and you become completely turned around, and you cannot recall how to get there. This is a typical symptom as one may lose spatial and visual perception, as well as directional challenges.

I believe many people whom are affected actually know before a family member. They realize their memory has radically changed from what they once recalled. Typically, you can expect doctors to direct questions to your loved one experiencing the changes and someone who lives in the home, generally a spouse. They are trying to capture an accurate picture of what is going on. People with dementia are not always aware of their condition. Therefore, it is essential your loved one never goes to their appointments alone.

Your primary care physician will likely make arrangements with a neurologist for testing. Because there is no single test that will determine dementia, many test are given to rule out what it is not and hopefully come up with a diagnosis. Test includes but they are not limited to cognitive assessments such as SLUMS or MoCA, neurological (checking balance, reflex, eye movement, and the like), lab work, brain scans (CT, MRI, PET), determining if one has sleep apnea, and an evaluation by a psychologist and/or a psychiatrist. This may be a little discouraging knowing the testing takes time. This is a process, and it takes time, sometimes months to have a diagnosis. Remember, you are trying to understand what is going on medically with your loved one. So much will transpire from the onset of the symptoms until you finally see your primary care doctor. Journaling (write) what you are experiencing in your home is beneficial. Note specific behaviors, instances, and stressors. Also know all medications your loved one is taking.

If your family has a history of dementia, one is possibly placed in a higher risk of developing the condition. There are some families with a family history that never experience symptoms and other families that do not have a history and experience symptoms. Fortunately, tests exist that can determine certain genetic mutations. However, the Alzheimer's Association and I concur; genes are only part of the picture. Whatever genes you have inherited, most people can significantly reduce their chances of getting dementia through simple lifestyle choices.

An article/study published by Nature Medicine in January 2019, stated researchers found a blood test could detect Alzheimer's up to 16 years before symptoms. Researchers believe by measuring changes in the levels of a protein in the blood may uncover early detection. This protein is called neurofilament light chain and if there is any rise in levels of the protein; it could be an early sign of the disease. Neurofilament light chain is a "marker in the blood which gives an indication of nerve cell loss in the brain," according to researcher Jucker, professor of cell biology of neurological diseases at the German Center for Neurodegenerative Diseases. The more neurofilament you have in the blood, the more brain damage you have he said. This new blood test will be "very important for clinical studies." He hopes the test will allow researchers to monitor the effectiveness of new treatments before people have started to experience symptoms, by measuring how levels of the protein are affected." The development of biomarkers for Alzheimer's disease is making it possible to detect Alzheimer's disease and provide accurate diagnosis earlier than at any

other time in history according to the
Alzheimer's Association. (Jucker, 2019,
p. 1–4)

What is a biomarker? A biomarker or biological
marker is a measurable indicator of some biological
state or condition. Biomarkers are often measured
and evaluated to examine normal biological processes,
pathogenic processes, or pharmacologic responses to a
therapeutic intervention.

In addition to providing significant medical,
emotional, social benefits, and facilitating participation
in important clinical trials; early diagnosis enables
individuals to prepare legal, financial, and end-of-life
plans. This is essential while your loved one is cognitively
able to make decisions and express their wishes.
This may sound daunting or morbid, but there is an inner
peace that will inevitably provide solace in lifestyle/estate
planning.

Caregiver Challenges

According to Alzheimer's Association 2020 Facts and Figures, there are more than sixteen million unpaid caregivers in the United States caring for their loved one who has one of the dementias. As previously discussed, Alzheimer's being at the top of the list for sufferers. The daunting task of a caregiver is unrelenting. Although the responsibilities have not waivered, resources are abundant. You are not alone! That refrain may sound rhetorical. More often than not, you may feel alone; it is vital to recognize that taking care of a loved one is a humongous commission. Therefore, it is imperative to discuss the challenges of this obligation because they are real.

The Center to Advance Palliative Care and the Gary and Mary West Health Institute teamed up to conduct four in-person focus groups and a survey of over five hundred caregivers to better understand what they contend with from their loved ones. While the research specifically addressed Alzheimer's, some of these behaviors you may find reflective in your home.

Caregivers noted the *most* challenging behaviors from their loved one included: agitation or aggression, repetitive speech or actions, wandering or restlessness,

incontinence and constipation.
Caregivers stated their challenges
included: dealing with memory loss,
impact of the disease on their loved one,
handling the stress and emotional toll
on oneself, patience, and coping with
the mood swings or behavioral changes.
(Sauer, 2018, p. 1–5)

Perhaps these are concerns that have manifested in your home. What are you to do? Your point of reference must always be to separate the disease from your loved one. What do I mean? When something happens, ask yourself, "Is this the disease or my loved one?" For example, your loved one, who would never use a profane word but now communicates effortlessly with profanity. You must immediately recognize that the disease is manifesting.

This is no fault of your loved one or you. It is the disease that you are witnessing. Try not to get upset, frustrated, or impatient. Redirecting the behavior is encouraged. I have said this before but try to live in their world as long as it is not detrimental to you or your loved one. You will find, especially in the onset of dementia, that your loved one may come across as though nothing is wrong around others. Has that happen to you? When family or friends are in their presence, they act quite convincing.

However, once company has departed, all the wheels on the wagon fall off. Why? In the earlier stages, they are able to masquerade very effectively because they know it is only for a short period of time. They are able to superficially maneuver settings that do not require in-depth cognition. Once they return home or guests leave your home, they return to behaviors that you prefer not to experience. That is because they know on some level their loved one will be there for them and sometimes they act most horribly with their loved one. Again, it hurts, and it is difficult, but your loved one would not intentionally seek to hurt you. They may also exhibit no filters and may cause you embarrassment.

Forget about trying to rationalize with your loved one. This will cause utter frustration on your behalf. Often times, this ability is no longer a part of your loved one's repertoire. They can no longer connect the dots. It does not matter the logic of your position, for them it is illogical, and you will not be able to convince them otherwise. I am sure you may be thinking, "This makes all the sense in the world," but not to your loved one. This could lead to an argument if you insist as you seek to be logical and/or prove a point. Let it go!

To reduce frustration, try to not request something of your loved one to do because they will inevitably forget. If your loved one really likes coffee and has a tendency to leave the pot on after usage, don't say to your loved one, "Honey, try and remember to cut off the pot." Just purchase a pot that has an automatic shut off. Again it keeps down the frustration for the both of you.

Are you thinking about Post-it notes? Initially they may work, but eventually they will forget to read them.

You must also be honest with yourself. However, therapeutic lying to your loved one is highly recommended. Dementia denotes memory lost. Does it really matter if your loved one thought their vehicle was a stick shift versus standard shift? It is not worth the confrontation. Your loved one will confuse dates, people, times, activities, and the like. Let it be because it can lead to distress for the both of you if you seek to correct or become brutally honest.

As a caregiver, have you found it difficult to express to the doctor what is really going on in your home? Often when you begin listing things your loved one is doing at home, they become angry. Possibly in their mind, they are thinking they have done none of the things described. It could lead to an argument or even your feelings being hurt. I know you just want the doctor to know what is going on in your home. We know when they are better helped, so is the caregiver. Hence, you must share with the doctor(s) all of the things that are occurring in the home as your loved one usually does not remember. To avoid confrontations, ask your doctor if you may submit in written format a week before the appointment; all of the things that are going on in the home. I have never known a doctor to say no to this request as they know the rationale behind the request. This provides the doctor insight, and it disallows an opportunity for your loved one to lash out at you. Suggestion, say one or two things from the letter to show you are engaged when the doctor is talking to the two of you during your office visit. Your letter writing may only serve as a temporary solution.

Try to refrain from so many questions. This takes practice because for so long, it was natural to ask questions. Often that is how conversations are ensued. Not anymore! If you are finding that no matter what you ask, your loved one poses the question back to you. They may not have the words and/or the ability to convey those words to you. Learn to make statements short in words and direct. Try hard to not be convoluted. For example, get to the point, do not expect a Freudian response, do not be disappointed with the response, and by all means, if the answer is not coherent, let it go!

As a caregiver, you are constantly juggling. Will you drop the balls? Yes! You cannot do it all, and you will not do it perfectly. Your loved one will remind you of that, and it is okay. You will experience a wide spectrum of emotions. If you are at your wits' end, you have hung in there too long without a break. You will need breaks. For some, it is weekly, and for others, it is monthly or quarterly. Please do not get caught up with quantity (how many times you need a break) but focus on quality. Your breaks provide quality care upon your return for your loved one.

You will absolutely need a support group. People you can count on that love the two of you. Individuals willing to step in for a couple of hours so you may experience a massage, pedicure, or a hairstyling appointment. If you are a male caregiver, perhaps fishing, hunting, or heading to the gym is your thing.

Maybe you want to walk the shoreline, take in a movie, or just hang out with your friends. These things are okay, but you need dependable people to ensure these quick breaks for you. Perhaps you have only shared your loved one's condition with a handful of people, that is fine. Your goal is to make sure they are dependable and have some basic knowledge/insight of your loved one's condition. The last thing you want is to have someone in your support circle taken aback by some of the behaviors of your loved one. Share basic tenants of your loved one's condition. It is also delightful for your loved one to get out. Let someone take them on a country ride on a sunshiny day or walk in the park. Develop a committed circle to help you navigate the quality care your loved one so deserves.

Attending support groups may also be gratifying for caregivers. You may gain new insight, meet new friends, or just being around others that relate to you because of the shared commonalty. Many find great comfort in being around others whom you do not have to explain the symptoms of the disease. Support groups are all around you and welcoming for you to attend.

Generally speaking, your loved one will have times when they are spot on. You will smile because you are in the present with your loved one, and it is inspiring. They will have moments of lucidity, that is to say, there will be times when they make sense and respond appropriately. Sadly I must share with you, this will not last. Some may think your loved one turns it on and off at will. Think about that for only a second, who would want to turn dementia on and off? When your loved one does manifest his or herself, through it all, treasure it all.

Each day is different and comes with a different set of circumstances. This will prove to be overwhelming and exhausting. Dementia is the inability to carry out everyday task as a consequence of diminished cognitive (thinking) abilities. As time passes and the disease worsens, I implore you to not allow it to get the best of you. Research illustrates that it can affect your health, your finances, your family, and your mental, emotional, and spiritual state. Dementia must be defeated. If it takes longer than we anticipate, we cannot and will not let it defeat us. Take care of yourself. All caregivers need breaks regularly as they cope with this catastrophic disease.

Adult Children Coping with their Parent's Dementia

It is difficult for adult children to witness the health decline of one or both of their parents. Most adult children know inevitably their parents are going to age. They may anticipate aging conditions such as hearing loss, vision impairment, and hip or knee replacement. But the diagnosis of one of the dementias is certainly a family game changer.

Typically, adult children no longer live at home. In fact, many have begun their own families and have full and busy lives. This generally leaves the parents with what one would refer to as an "empty nest." Most parents look forward to having their home and lives to one another with the hopes of actually completing some of their bucket list activities such as retirement, travel, and leisure. Then one of the parents becomes stricken with an illness. For the adult child who has to cope with a dementia diagnosis, it is family altering.

The mere processing of having your parent virtually diminishing before your eyes is heart wrenching. They look exactly the same, but adult children eventually see and hear the decline, especially if you live close to one another. Logistically, if you do not live close by, it is often hard to detect dementia. On the phone or during Facetime, they seem quite the same. However, keep in mind in the early and midrange of dementia, your loved one can masquerade quite well. Why? You are on the phone for a brief time, and conversation is light and airy and fun engagement. They manage through these brief periods. However, bear in mind, once you hang up the phone, they return to the emotional and physical effects of the disease. The caregiver is the one who receives all of the residuals of the disease. You are encouraged to not be bamboozled into thinking your caregiver mom or dad is making things up or exaggerating the circumstances. They are not!

Generally speaking, adult children do not immediately grasp the concept that their parent is slowly but surely losing their independence, personality, and characteristics. This is a difficult transition for adult children to watch a parent slip away. After all, this is the individual that hopefully impacted their life the most.

However, your otherwise vibrant parent will eventually need your caregiving attention, and as time elapses, it will be evident. Simply put, your other parent *cannot* carry the full responsibility of the parent with dementia. I am optimistically thinking, you will want to assist in an impactful manner.

As adult children, you may not immediately come into the full understanding of what a dementia diagnosis means. You will need to process yourself through a couple of significant areas. These areas include denial, anger, guilt, sadness, and acceptance (Clarity Point, 2018). You will get there! Let us examine each of these areas.

- *Denial.* You may think caregiver mom/dad is just exaggerating. It cannot be that bad. After all, he/she sounds/seems great on the phone or in person. You may even dupe yourself into thinking it will get better. It does not.
- *Anger.* Once you have worked through the denial process, anger may set in. This is an okay emotion. You are mad and may ask why? You are mad because there will be family changes for sure. You are encouraged to work through the anger as it will liberate you.
- *Guilt.* You may feel guilty because eventually you will not be able to connect with your loved, and you will want to. You will get beyond this because it may not be the traditional method of connecting, but you will find your unique way to reach your loved one.
- *Sadness.* You will experience great sadness because you are processing loss. It is perfectly natural that your interactions with your loved one will cause you sadness. Hopefully, it will come and go. If you need professional help, seek it. Do not get stuck in sadness.
- *Acceptance.* You will get here. At this point, you will empower yourself by educating yourself with information on the disease. You will develop special ways to connect with your loved. *Always* give support and encouragement to your caregiver mom/dad (Clarity Pointe, 2018, p. 1–7)

The grieving process is just that, a process. There is no specific timeline; it is just important to get through the emotional process. A couple of final coping techniques. Again process your emotions. Find someone who will listen to you and be able to empathize with you. Do not let your family circumstances capture and leave you in emotional turmoil. You will need support. Reach out because help is all around you.

If you have to eventually become a caregiver, do the very best you can. You must take breaks away from your loved one to rejuvenate. Take good care of yourself, exercise, eat healthy, refrain from smoking and drinking as much as possible. Interestingly enough, these are also great habits that disrupt dementia and certainly promote brain health.

Legal Plans

I must preface this conversation by noting every
state has different laws, and laws do change. You must
consult with an attorney, preferable an elder care attorney
representing your state for the care of your loved one's
estate. The information I am about to provide is generic/
basic and must be tailored to your family.

According to the Alzheimer's Association, there are
four areas of concern. They are as follows: legal capacity,
legal documents, finding an attorney, and meeting
with your attorney. Let us now extrapolate on each.
Legal capacity, if your loved one has the capacity to
understand the significance of having legal documents
in place, they perhaps have the legal capacity/ability
to understand and thereby sign documents. If you are
unsure, an attorney can help you determine what level of
legal capacity is required for your loved one to sign any
legal documents. The Alzheimer's Association suggests
you talk with your loved one to confirm what is being
explained and what is being asked of your loved one.
Their doctor can also lend their expertise as to whether
or not your loved one understands. If your loved one has
developed legal documents pre-dementia diagnosis, it
would be wise to review the said documents and make

necessary corrections and/or updates. I personally would seek an attorney because I know education, not law.

Legal Documents, such as: Living
Will, Living Trust, Power of Attorney,
Power of Attorney for Health Care,
or Guardianship/Conservatorship.
If you are a military family, it may
be prudent to reach out to see if the
military requires any additional legal
documents. Many legal documents can
be obtained and completed without the
assistance of an attorney. If you decide
to seek an attorney for advice and or
services, seek one that specializes in Elder
Care Law. The Alzheimer's Association
suggestions: If you have an attorney in
the family or an attorney friend, they
may be able to refer you to someone.
The Alzheimer's Association has a list of
elder law attorneys in your area. Their
24 hour a day/7 days a week telephone
number is: 800 272-3900. Contact
your local Area Agency on Aging or the
Eldercare locator at 800 677-1116 or
visit eldercare.gov for free legal resources.
Meeting with an attorney, discuss all of
your concerns and prepare questions
prior to your visit. You definitely want to
know options for health and long term

care, options for managing personal care
and property, and possible coverage of
long-term care services, including what
is provided by Medicare, Medicaid, and
certainly Veteran benefits and any other
long term care insurance in your state.
Furthermore, the Alzheimer's Association
additionally recommends that those
couples who are not in legally recognized
relationships are especially vulnerable
to limitations regarding the ability to
make decisions for each other and may
be unable to obtain information about a
partner's health status if legal documents
are not completed. Laws vary from state
to state; make sure you understand
your state's laws and your rights.
The Alzheimer's Association has brochure
entitled "LGBT Caregiver Concerns."
You may download this information by
going to their website or call their 800
number. (Alzheimer's Association, 2014,
p. 1–10)

Again, I am a long-time educator, not an attorney.
However, I introduced you to my grandmother much
earlier in this book; she always thought I should have
gone to law school. Ha! One day, remind me to share that
story.

Clinical Trials

As an advocate for dementia, I must admit that in addition to my activism, I am vitally concerned with minorities and the alarming effects of one of the dementias destroying our communities. To preserve brain health, expedite a cure; we must be involved with clinical trials.

If you have been affected by Alzheimer's, Dementia, or Mild Cognitive Impairment, there is something you— and only people like you—can do to help find a cure: participate in a clinical trial. Your body may hold the answers to medical researchers' questions about the disease. If you're in a clinical trial, you're part of the research team working to find ways to prevent Alzheimer's. Why Clinical Trials? They look at new ways to detect, prevent, or cure diseases. Often, people who participate in clinical trials learn more about their own condition from medical experts using advanced technology. Sometimes, participants are the first people to benefit

> from a new treatment. Trials are designed
> to be safe and as convenient as possible.
> (Us Against Alzheimer's, 2014, p. 1–8)

If you are Black, you are probably thinking, "I don't trust the medical profession with trials and studies." I understand your apprehension as a Black woman. I know all too well studies like the Tuskegee Syphilis Study and countless other morally repugnant, deplorable, and unconscionable studies. I get it. However, as of this writing, Blacks, Latinos, and Hispanics are the three leading races suffering from Alzheimer's disease (may have begun as dementia). Moreover, we are also the racial groups with the least participation in clinical trials. Trials help exert power over the disease, embrace hope for the future, and ultimately help find treatment and cures according to Us Against Alzheimer's. Honestly writing, the medical profession needs us to find a cure, and we need them to find a cure.

> Are Clinical Trials safe now? Researchers
> want their trials to be safe. They also
> are required to follow strict rules
> to make sure participants are safe.
> Trials in the United States are approved
> and monitored by a committee of
> doctors, scientists, and other people
> with expertise in research ethics and law.
> This is known as the Institutional Review
> Board (IRB). It is designed to ensure the

risks are reduced and are outweighed by potential benefits. The IRB reviews the trial before it starts and as it proceeds to protect participants' rights and safety. During any trial, a participant has the right to stop the trial at any time. Today, many clinical trials for Alzheimer's disease prefers the participant to have what is called a study partner. This person generally is a caregiver or someone close to the participant. Their responsibility is to assist the participant through the process with things such as transportation for participation, reminders of appointments, encourages the participant, and provides information which helps to determine the success of the clinical trial. In a nutshell, what is the process to participate? Contact a clinical research center (ADEAR) can assist you. They will conduct a prescreening to ensure you meet the criteria for the trial. Sometimes they look for specific genders, age, medical history, or even race. There are thousands of clinical trials that take place across the nation. Remember, they need us to participate. Further diagnostic screening is necessary to determine who will continue with the trial. You will be admitted into the

trial and receive the medical treatment
or a placebo, researchers will monitor
the effects. At the end of the clinical
trial, many studies reduce greatly the
monitoring of your health thereafter.
There are two types of proteins that
cause brain cells to stop functioning,
lose connections with other brain cells,
and die. (A) Amyloid plaques build up
over time and interrupt the messages
conducted from one part of the brain
to another. (B) Neurofibrillary tangles
are snarls of proteins that systematically
destroy brain cells from the inside.
(Us Against Alzheimer's, 2019, p. 1–8)

Clinical trials promote early detection and treatment.
It improves patient care for a longer period of time
and allows families to strategically plan their finances.
As I encourage clinical trials, I want to conclude by
sharing an African proverb: "If you want to go fast, go
alone but if you want to go far go together." They need
us, and we need them.

I have retweeted, and it is worth repeating again.
According to Us Against Alzheimer's, "The fact of the
matter is; the first person to be cured of Alzheimer's will
be in a clinical trial."

What Not to Say and a Few More Facts

In 2017, the Alzheimer's Society's blog offered seven suggestions on what *not* to say to someone with dementia.

1. Remember when…
2. I just told you that…
3. Your brother died ten years ago…
4. What did you do this morning…
5. Do you recognize me…
6. Let's have a cup of tea now, then we can go for a nice walk and get lunch at the café in town…
7. Do you need some help with that, love?

My suggestions when dealing with the seven aforementioned tenants discussed by the Alzheimer's Society.

1. This time last year, we were at the lake…try not to ask but suggest/tell.
2. It seems to me, no matter how you say this, it sounds rude. A good practice is to just say it again as though it is your first time.
3. I do not believe the topic of death is relevant to them. It may conjure pain or confusion. If you must share be sensitive and keep it simple.

A recent observation. A dementia patient was told her daughter had passed away. She laughed and said she was happy because she was eating shrimp and fish.

4. Too many questions cause stress. Due to their inability to come up with words and articulate their thoughts.

5. There is a probability they may not know who you are. This is acceptable. Do not make them feel guilty. In all stages of dementia, a simple hello is good.

6. It is difficult to process run-on sentences as an English teacher would say. Give one suggestion at a time, no yelling in crowds, and make sure you have their undivided attention.

7. Pet names can be annoying! Just call the person with dementia by their name. Not only does this reinforce who they are as an individual; it speaks to their humanity.

Additional information on statement number five from the Dementia & Alzheimer's Wellbeing Network better known as DAWN.

There are a number of reasons that people with dementia can "forget" even their closest family members. Dementia affects the part of the brain that enables recognition of features and familiarity in human faces. They suggest the most

important thing is to avoid reacting
with concern or hurt. The inability
to recognize loved ones is part of
experiencing dementia. Grieve in private,
but respond to your loved one with calm
acceptance or redirection. If redirection
does not work, just accept the mistaken
identity. (Blog Post, 2019)

I concur, again it does hurt, but they are not
purposely trying to hurt you. Let it go. Do not be
insistent that they must know who you are. Honestly, they
probably just don't know who you are.

A few more 2019 facts and figures from Us Against
Alzheimer's.

- Women are twice as likely as men to develop
  Alzheimer's.
- Latinos are 1.5 times more likely to have
  Alzheimer's than Whites, and by 2060, the
  number of Latinos in the United States living
  with Alzheimer's is expected to be 3.5 million.
- Blacks are two to three times more likely to
  develop Alzheimer's than other populations.
- Veterans who have suffered traumatic brain
  injuries are 60 percent more likely to develop
  Alzheimer's.

Dementia and Driving

Losing the independence driving provides can be upsetting. It is important to acknowledge a person's feelings and preserve his or her independence, while ensuring the person's safety and the safety of others according to the Alzheimer's Association 2018.

This conversation is not always an easy one. Below are some tips on starting the conversation of driving and what to do when the conversation does not go so well.

> Initiate a dialogue to express your concerns. Address resistance while reaffirming your love and support. Appeal to your loved ones sense of responsibility. Reinforce medical diagnoses and directives. Ask the physician to write a letter stating your loved one cannot drive. Or ask the physician to write a prescription that says "No driving." You can then use the letter or prescription to reinforce the conversation. Consider an evaluation by an objective party. Understand that this may be the first of many conversations

about driving. Some people will give up driving easily but for others it could be difficult. Be prepared for the person to become angry with you. This may be their last hope of independence and they may be reluctant to give up the keys. Be patient and firm but display understanding and empathy. Acknowledge the pain of this change and appeal again to their sense of responsibilities. Ask a respected family authority figure to reinforce the message about not driving. Do not blame yourself if it does not go well. (Alzheimer's Association, 2018, p. 1–5)

How do you know when it is time to hide the keys? Will you know when it has become unsafe? Yes, absolutely. What will you observe?

- Forgetting where familiar places are located in your city.
- Becoming confused when driving, especially when the signage is good
- Confusing the break and the gas pedal.
- Speeding, excessive lane changes, and staring straight ahead.
- Taking a lot longer than the average time to reach a destination.

- Returning to a familiar city/place, i.e., parents home but turned around directionally.

Dementia changes your loved one's perception of things. As previously discussed, it impairs their thinking, reasoning, and judgement. Please do not expect them to have a rational conversation about their inability to drive. Not likely. Encourage them by offering other modes of transportation such as Uber, Lyft, or special transportation services in your community. Of course you would facilitate those travels. Try to think ahead in terms of minimizing their having to drive. Grocery shop in advance, use delivery services, or arrange rides to appointments. Plan ahead for this conversation because there will come a day when it will be necessary. This is another hard subject to deal with because you do not want anything to happen to your loved one, nor do you want anything to happen to anyone else on the road.

Legislation and Research

Congress heard the clarion call to join the campaign against Alzheimer's disease, according to the Alzheimer's Association. On December 31, 2018, the Alzheimer's Association and the Alzheimer's Impact Movement (AIM) are celebrating the passage of the Building Our Largest Dementia (BOLD) infrastructure for Alzheimer's Act which was signed into law on the aforementioned date. The law will enhance and improve our nation's public health response to the Alzheimer's crisis and further demonstrate that the 115th Congress remains fully committed to the fight to end Alzheimer's.

It was stated, 5 million Americans are living with the disease and by 2050; this number is projected to rise to nearly 14 million. It is the most expensive disease in the country costing an estimated $277 billion including $186 billion in direct costs to Medicare and Medicaid in 2018. Chief Public Policy Officer, Robert Egge was quoted as saying "Thanks to all the elected officials who championed this legislation, the country will now be better able to

fight this devastating disease as we
continue to work towards our vision
of a world without Alzheimer's. As an
important point, this law was introduced
by Senators Susan Collins (Maine),
Catherine Cortez Masto (Nevada),
Shelley Moore Capito (West Virginia),
and Tim Kaine (Virginia). House
of Representatives Brett Guthrie
(Kentucky), Paul Tonko (New York),
Chris Smith (New Jersey) and Maxine
Waters (California). One of these
individuals may be your representative,
and you may want to acknowledge their
contribution to the cause. In addition,
more than half of Congress cosponsored
the bill but the above mentioned
names introduced the Alzheimer's Act.
(Alzheimer's Association, 2018, p. 1–3)

The University of Michigan led a
study that was published in The
American Heart Association's Journal
of Hypertension which suggest blood
pressure may help explain why black
adults who are more likely to develop
high blood pressure; also are two times
more likely to have dementia later in life.
The study also suggested that aggressively
treating high blood pressure could

reduce the risk of cognitive impairment in a wider population of older adults, particularly in Black adults and men. Dr. Deborah A. Levine, the study's lead author and an Associate Professor of Internal Medicine and Neurology at the University of Michigan Medical School further stated, "We currently don't have very effective treatments for dementia, so preventing it is crucial." The article entitled Blood Pressure May Explain Higher Dementia Risks in Blacks further stated the Brain is one of the main organs to feel the effects of hypertension. High Blood pressure alters blood vessels and makes it more likely for arteries to harden and narrow. If blood flow is ineffective to the brain, damage can occur that impacts cognitive ability. Cognitive Impairment and dementia (not Alzheimer's) affects 8.6 million Americans. This could triple by 2050, with associated cost at 1.1 trillion. The study according to Dr. Adolfo Correa, whom was not a part of the study, believes "The study provides more rationale for aggressive screening and treatment of hypertension. It is important to replicate findings and understand the reasons for the racial and ethnic and racial disparities in cognitive

impairment and high blood pressure."
(Health Day, 2019, p. 1–2)

Because Blacks are at risk, a study by Regenstrief Institute in April 2018 found that controlling blood pressure with medications can prevent dementia in older Blacks. According to the institute, they were able to find in their twenty-four-year study, substantial evidence that supports the taking of antihypertension medicine (generic medicine is effective) may reduce the onset of dementia in sixty-five and older blacks.

In previous work by Regenstrief Institute, researchers reported that antihypertensive medication had a protective effect, reducing the odds of cognitive impairment in older African Americans. The new study investigated the effect of antihypertensive medications on cognitive impairment and dementia, determining that it is blood pressure reduction rather than the medications that lower the risk of dementia.
Per Dr. Michael Murray, "Controlling blood pressure is important for lowering the risk of heart attack, stroke and kidney disease, and now we can add the prevention of dementia to the list of benefits of good blood pressure control at all age. Preventing dementia is critical;

once you start the decline from cognitive
impairment to mild and eventually
severe dementia there is no known cure."
(Scientific Daily, 2018, p. 1–5)

Emory University in Georgia expresses their position
by literally discussing a piece that was written entitled
"The Heart of the Matter." The heart has been proven to
be a key component in the rise of African Americans and
Alzheimer's.

The heart pumps around one-fifth of
blood to the brain. This blood provides
essential nutrients and oxygen to the
body's brain cells allowing the brain to
thrive and function normally. Dr. Monica
Parker, MD and Assistant Professor
of Medicine of the Department of
Neurology of Emory Alzheimer's Disease
Research Center states "Higher rates of
cardiovascular diseases, hypertension
and diabetes, in these groups increases
risk of stroke, a key risk factor for
cognitive dysfunction related to vascular
dementia." High blood pressure, diabetes,
and high cholesterol damage the heart
and make it very difficult to transport
all of those nutrients to your entire body
including the brain. This lack of oxygen
affects brain functions like speech and

memory. Obviously according to the
Healthy Aging article, some factors
cannot be avoided like age and family
illnesses. (Emory University, 2016,
p. 1–4)

Note, dementia is not a normal part of aging, and dementia can occur in younger people. However, there are many factors we can maintain. Factors such as our weight, blood pressure, blood sugar, and cholesterol should be maintained by a healthy lifestyle. Moreover, regular checkups to possibly eradicate and/or minimize any of the dementias is highly encouraged. Dementia is not a specific disease. Instead, dementia describes a group of symptoms affecting memory, thinking, and social abilities severely enough to interfere with daily functioning. Hence, cognitive, psychological, and social changes are impacted.

According to Salud America, a national Latino-focused organization. It creates culturally relevant and research based stories and tools to inspire people to drive healthy changes to policies, systems, and environments for Latino children and families. This organization operationally defined the bill's provisions regarding detection and treatment and access to care.

Detection and Treatment: The bill
"directs the Centers for Medicare
and Medicaid Services to require use

of Cognitive Impairment detection tool or set of tools identified by the National Institutes of Health. Use of these tools will incentivize clinicians to detect and diagnose Alzheimer's and related dementias in their earliest stages. If cognitive impairment is detected, patients are to be referred for additional testing, to community-based support services, and to appropriate clinical trials." What is more, Access to Care: the bill "Requires the Centers of Medicare and Medicaid Services to lead, create, adopt, and recognize quality measures and incentives to promote the detection and diagnosis of Alzheimer's or related dementias and appropriate care planning services, including potential for clinical trial participation." The Center for Disease Control indicates the total number of Alzheimer's cases will rise from 4.9 million in 2014 to 1.4 billion in 2060, adversely affecting Blacks and Latinos. (Salud America, 2019, p. 1–7)

The acronym CHANGE stands for Concentrating on High-Value Alzheimer's Needs to Get to an End. This Act brought forth in the 115th Congress in 2018, promotes early detection of cognitive impairment, increased access to appropriate care for people with Alzheimer's disease. It also aims its efforts to keep individuals in their communities and provide caregivers with financial assistance and certification. The status of the legislation is as follows: The House of Representatives introduced the bill (number 4957) in February 7, 2018, and referred it to the subcommittee on Health and the Committee on Ways and Means on February 13, 2018.

It was also referred to the Subcommittee on Health in the Committee on Energy and Commerce on February 9, 2018. The senate (number 2387) introduced the bill on February 7, 2018. It was read twice and referred to the committee on finance.

The act was reintroduced April 2019 to gain more traction as there are so many new faces in the 116th Congress and introduced a bit earlier in the year to affect change. This is a good start.

In 2018, American Association of Retired People (AARP) and Fleishman Hillard Global Intelligence conducted an online survey polling five hundred doctors for their perspective of dementia. The survey was not the most hopeful but revealing it was. Nearly half of those surveyed (49 percent) stated dementia is a hopeless diagnosis today and forty-seven percent stated they prefer their patients to introduce the subject during their visit. They admit they have little to offer.

The juxtaposition of another survey conducted by AARP researchers illustrates the importance of education on the topic of dementia and brain health. Why? Nearly half of the participants believe treatment existed to stop the progress of Alzheimer's. And two out of three of the participants believe Alzheimer's can be diagnosed with a single test. As the reader of my book, I know, you already knew the correct answers. Of course you did!

A majority of those surveyed (59 percent) think that Alzheimer's is a mental illness, and three-quarters (75 percent) think that memory loss is a normal and natural part of aging. Although it is normal for aging adults to forget a name or date, this type of information is typically recalled later. It is not normal, to forget where you live. There are so many myths and misconceptions about the aging brain. That is even more true when you are talking about dementia, said Sarah Lock, AARP senior vice president for policy and executive director of the Global Council on Brain Health. Although almost everyone knows dementia is a serious problem for families, our research shows health care professionals as well as consumers need more information and education to better address the problem. With few educational, diagnostic or healing tools at their disposal, physicians often bypass opportunities to evaluate patients for dementia. Most respondents in the AARP Research survey (63%) stated they have never been asked about

their cognition during a routine checkup.
(AARP, 2018, p. 2–3)

Caregivers, you are the strongest advocate for your loved one and at the earliest possible stage of detection. None of us can wait around until our physician asks us about our brain health. We need to request brain health assessments as a part of our annual checkups when seen by our doctor. Empowering ourselves with education for our family is a must. Knowledge and access is power!

Train the Author and Consensus Building

You have managed to continue reading this book, and I am humbled and certainly thankful. At this point, I wish to share scenarios with you. I want you to respond in writing based on your reading and knowledge from the book or your own experience. There are no wrong or right answers. Here we go…

1. Your great uncle was diagnosed with Alzheimer's, and he lives in a neighboring state. You have been told he is very difficult to deal with and has a weapon. You are particularly fond of this uncle, so you drive over to do a wellbeing check. Initially the visit begins well, not too much time into the visit, he becomes loud, belligerent, threatening, and accusatory. What is your response?

____

____

____

____

____

____

2. Your good friend was delightful, articulate, caring, smart, and a community activist. You have known her well over a decade, and you guys generally intersect with community service projects. You run into her, and you are met with a quizzical look as though she does not know you. How do you respond?

____

____

____

____

____

____

____

3. Last year, you and a sister from the church were discussing the possibility of volunteering for VBS (Vacation Bible School). While not intimate with one another in terms of phone conversations, day trips, luncheons, and the like, you guys know each other from church. You see her nine months later, and she smiles at you but without the warm embrace as in the past. How do you react?

____

____

____

____

____

____

____

4. Your husband has dementia. You visit your daughter in another state for two weeks. This is the longest time you have been away since his diagnosis. He states to other family members while you are away traveling that he does not miss you. However, immediately upon your return, he says to you, "You know I am sick. You should not have left me." What do you say to your husband? Will you leave again for a getaway?

____

____

____

____

____

____

5. Your mom has dementia. She is living with you for several months. You are really clean and neat. Your mom is the antithesis. You watch her make a mess, and you ask her, "Why didn't you clean up your mess?" She retorts, "I did not make that mess!" How do you respond to your mom?

____

____

____

____

____

____

6. Your husband has reached his plateau on his current dementia medication. He needs a higher dosage than his current meds. How would you know this?

____

____

____

____

____

____

7. Follow on from question 6. Your husband is refusing to go to the next higher dosage of medication because he says it makes him sick after two days of trying it. How will you get your husband to the next higher dosage prescribed by his doctor?

____

____

____

____

____

____

8. Your wife who is on medication for dementia symptoms was hospitalized for a medical procedure. The nurse comes in to dispense medication. As he goes over the medication that he brought in, he is unfamiliar with one of the meds, and it is your wife's medication for her symptoms. He asks, "What is this medication for?" What do you say?

____

____

____

____

____

____

9. Your friend's husband displays all the classical signs of dementia. He has a diagnosis and takes medication. She works full time, and he is mostly left to his on self-care throughout the day. Your friend comes home exhausted. He sings very well, loves music, and he wants to sing in his band. How will you handle this situation?

____

____

____

____

____

____

10. Your husband is on medication for dementia
    symptoms, and you have been coping with
    it for the past two years. You have completed
    many small things to compliment the home.
    Nothing major but noticeable in the home.
    Your husband says nothing about the many small
    home makeovers. Are your feeling hurt? How do
    you respond?

____

____

____

____

____

____

____

11. An associate you met at an educational social
    club where you presented a speech on Alzheimer's
    and other dementias pulls you to the side to
    discuss Alzheimer's. His mother was diagnosed.
    He obviously prefers to discuss the concern one
    on one. How do you respond?

____

____

____

____

____

____

12. Your wife has dementia with several functionalities. However, she comes home with a new car that she has purchased. While your wife did broach the subject with you, there was no meeting of the minds. Your other vehicles are operating just fine. How will you respond?

____

____

____

____

____

____

13. Your husband is on medication for dementia symptoms. This was the very first year on Mother's Day that he did nothing for you other than a card. How are you feeling? How would you respond?

____

____

____

____

____

____

14. Your husband with Alzheimer's has just struck you. He has never so much as said an unkind word to you. You told him you would throw something away if he did not keep an eye on it. That set him off. What should you have not done? How would you handle the situation after being struck in the face?

____

____

____

____

____

____

____

You have done well with this mini exercise. I would like to share with you my responses as these are real scenarios. Also real in the sense that you may have already dealt with similar circumstances or you may encounter them during your journey. Hopefully you will concur with my responses or you may have a better solution.

1. Due to the threatening manner, it is best to exit immediately. Again, you never want to place yourself and/or remain in a dangerous situation. Try to get your loved one help from a distance.
2. I would not ask, "Do you remember me?" I would smile and move on gracefully.

Clearly something is going on as that was not her typical response toward you.

3. Smile and keep it moving. She does not know who you are at that moment and perhaps never again.

4. Smile and share how much you have missed him and how glad you are to be home with him. Reassure, reassure. Indeed, you will take another caregiver's break, but that topic does not call for a conversation.

5. *In her mind,* she did not make the mess. I can see why she feels as though she shouldn't have to clean it up. Do not go back and forth with her. In fact, when there is a mess, just clean it up. Or say, "Would you like to help me clean up?" She may say no, so expect that too. Do not major in the minor.

6. Simply by paying attention to the symptoms/ behaviors. Symptoms are always present, but when off the medication or if the medication is ineffective, the symptoms are magnified. Pay attention!

7. Through encouragement, coaxing, reassuring, and creating an environment by which one feels supported. Seek the assistance of your doctor to encourage your loved one. This is a bit more challenging when your loved one has degrees of functionality. Try to catch them in a space of lucidity to encourage the higher dose.

8. Answer the question and, if you can, use
    the conversation as a teachable moment.
    Many caregivers will take their loved one
    off of their medicine without the opinion of
    the doctor. Many will say it is not doing any
    good. Some medications work better than
    others for people with Alzheimer's or one of
    the other dementias. I say consider tweaking
    the medication until one shows some affect.
    Medication is not a cure all. It simply minimizes
    the symptoms that you see and experience.
    We must continue the fight because there is no
    cure as I write. What is the fight? More money
    for research and fight against financial
    congressional cuts.
9. Share with her gently that it is likely he will
    not remember the words of the song. If he is
    insistent, inform the band and maybe they can
    do something with him inclusively by which he
    could sing. In addition, allow music to be a part
    of his daily life. I also suggest the Music Memory
    Box. Research points to the fact that individuals
    with dementia absolutely love music.
10. Yes, your feelings may be hurt. Understand that
    your husband as you once knew him would have
    commented on the special things you did to
    beautify the home. Differentiate the disease from
    your husband. This will disallow your feeling
    overly sensitive when he/she makes no comment.
    I am inclined to believe they may have noticed

but did not have words to convey what it means to them. Keep doing the small things but do not depend upon your loved one to say kudos. A friend or family remember will notice, and they will compliment you. Accept and appreciate their recognition of your talent. I know you want your loved one to do it, but he/she are no longer in that place. Do not set yourself up for disappointment by being let down when your loved one seems to not acknowledge and/or appreciate your deeds. Their lack of apathy and/or empathy is real.

11. Great! You have an opportunity to share your knowledge and/or resources. Encouragement is key because this is a hard disease. Imagine your inability to connect with your mom of all people. According to Mary McLeod Bethune, "Next to God, we are indebted to women, first for life itself, and then for making it worth living."

12. You have to be awfully persuasive at this point. Rationalization is often met with opposition as they cannot connect the dots. Hence, your gentle persuasiveness must come in handy. Hopefully, you have been building bridges along the way so you can have some influence. Often they struggle with expenses, finances, and what is logical. Sometimes they are preyed upon because they have the inability to make sound financial decisions, and people take advantage. They often spend quite a bit of money if they

have access because they have no concept of its value. If push comes to shove, you must then go to the car lot and speak with management. Always pray for favor.

13. Be thankful he remembered the card! You said it: "This was the first year he did nothing but a card." That is an indicator of the progression of the dementia. Reflect and smile upon on all of the wonderful things he did on past Mother's Days. I know this is hard but do not take it personal.

14. You do not have to have the last word. It generally comes across threatening and possibly invokes a confrontation. They can be unpredictable, but the last thing you want to do is come across provokingly. At this point, a caregiver getaway would be highly advised.

If you are wondering why several answers included "smile," it is because a smile is a universal language, and it conveys a sense of all is well. I am smiling now because you did well with this consensus building exercise.

My Revelation

The writing of this book has taught me the heartbreak of the disease but also the resilience of people involved in this quagmire. I am encouraged by all of the organizations, agencies, physicians, researchers, and caregivers. These individuals work hour by hour and day by day tirelessly to disrupt dementia. As of this writing, it is commonplace to encounter someone whose loved one has Alzheimer's or one of the other dementias. If in fact, it has not affected you directly, the odds are, it will likely affect you indirectly. Perhaps, a coworker, a friend, someone in your house of faith, in your social circle, or your neighbor may encounter one of the dementias. The disease is everywhere and leaving collateral damage all around us. Sadly there is no cure, and it is prevalent and pervasive.

I have four major takeaways after writing this book. Actually, there are several, but I will discuss the four most passionate revelations for me. First, research often negates populations that are in most need. Currently, it is Blacks, Hispanics, and Latinos. Seemingly, research is conducted with populations that are easy and convenient to enroll in studies.

This precludes the aforementioned populations in clinical trials and, therefore, disallows opportunities to medically determine the effects and/or impacts of treatment responses and prognosis on the aforementioned populations. Moreover, researchers must take seriously the importance of involving minorities in clinical trials. Health care practitioners, if patients cannot get to you, you must get to them. This would derail disparities and will open the doors to access.

What is more, conferences, workshops, and seminars must consider lowering their cost for inclusion/participation. Particularly if one is serious about educating and eradicating through prevention and intervention, inclusion is paramount. Why wouldn't one want to include the very populations who need the information most? Consider reducing your cost for attendance purposes or provide access by offering one-day free workshops in the communities of the aforementioned. Sponsorships to defray cost from the medical community and/or practitioners for this type of education would be plentiful.

Secondly, I taught government for over a decade, and I believe in the core values of this country. Our government needs to do more financially to support the research of this deadly disease called Alzheimer's and its related dementias. According to Us Against Alzheimer's 2019 reporting, for every dollar the federal government spends today on the costs of Alzheimer's care, it invests less than a penny in research to find a cure. Through research, a cure or treatment can be developed. It was done for other diseases such as tuberculosis and HIV/AIDS; it can be done again. Hold your elected officials accountable. Stigmas surrounding dementia may prevent individuals from participating in clinical trials that may lead to treatment and/or a diagnosis. Hence, more public awareness and understanding is necessary. Myths must be debunked; so families may walk, pardon me, race toward liberation. Monies from the federal government must be insisted upon to allocate toward research.

Third, we the people must assume responsibility for our brain health lifestyle. What is included in this lifestyle? Management of weight, hypertension (high blood pressure), diabetes, cholesterol, and excessive consumptions of alcohol are essential. We can also develop more of a plant-based diet, exercise, sleep, stay social, and partake in mentally stimulating activities that insist we critically think and analyze. Will these suggestions guarantee your not acquiring one of the dementias? There is no such guarantee. However, it potentially reduces your risk of one of the dementias and cognitive decline. At a bare minimum, the suggestions above should lead to a heathier lifestyle including brain health.

Fourthly, denial is powerful. It is very easy to deny what is going on before your very eyes with Alzheimer's and related dementias. While challenging, you must understand your loved one is dependent upon your activism. I recently heard a neurologist state he denied all the signs given to him by his mother concerning his dad. As a neurologist, his profession diagnose individuals with Alzheimer's and other dementias, but his denial hindered what was before his eyes in part because it was "dad." It is not unusual to blow off symptoms and say, "Oh, Mom/Dad will be okay. Everyone forgets their keys."

Yes, that may be correct, but when keys are forgotten several times a week, they lock themselves out of the house, they lock the keys in the car while the car is still running, and they cannot retrace keys, it calls for concern. You know your loved one, and you know their character. You may be the only family member willing to sacrifice and/or acknowledge the condition of Mom/Dad.

You cannot park in denial, put the car in drive because time is of the essence with this disease. Get the help you need because this disease and all the territory that goes along with it does not wait or get easier. If you are in denial, it is okay. There is no time like the present. Seek the help you need as it is abundantly available. God speed.

Finally, many opportunities have presented themselves that has allowed me to personally serve others by offering insight on dementia. While as complicated as the disease is, my desire is to help others better understand and cope with it. I also have learned the utter importance of ensuring minorities, such as I, become increasingly empowered with knowledge to achieve access. The disease is unrelenting and robs one of their dignity and their life as it was once known.

I am optimistic, a Believer, an advocate, and unyielding. During a recent webinar discussing brain health featuring Anne Tumlinson, she stated approximately 70 percent of individuals either fully or partially rely on their faith while coping with the disease. "But they that wait upon the Lord shall renew their strength; they shall mount up with wings as eagles; they shall run, and not be weary; and they shall walk, and not faint" (Isaiah 40:31).

The word *race* is used in the title of my book as a double entendre. Why? This is a race, and we must cross the finish line with a cure. While the book is relevant for each race, specific racial groups such as Blacks, Hispanics, and Latinos are disproportionately affected. Consequently, it is *the race of dementia.*

Glossary

AFB Air Force Base.

anosognosia It is a lack of ability to perceive the realities of one's own condition. It is a person's inability to accept that they have a condition that matches up with their symptoms or a formal diagnosis. It is a result of changes to the brain.

aphasia An inability or difficulty to formulating language, expressing one's thoughts and understanding another person's statements because of damage to specific brain regions.

cognition The act of knowing, including judgement and awareness.

computed tomography (CT) An X-ray technique that produces detailed, cross-sectional images of the head and body.

delusions Sustained false belief that something is true when it is not.

demented Never use the word to refer to someone with dementia. It is derogatory.

depression A condition characterized by loss of interest in normal daily activities. Feelings of sadness, helplessness, and/or hopelessness.

DNA (deoxyribonucleic acid) The carrier of genetic information.

dystonia Is a neurological movement disorder syndrome in which sustained or repetitive muscle contractions result in twisting and repetitive movements or abnormal fixed postures.

magnetic resonance imaging (MRI) A technique that uses a magnetic field and radio waves to create cross-sectional images of the head and body.

masked facies Loss of facial expressions.

mild cognitive impairment (MCI) Causes a slight but noticeable and measurable decline in cognitive abilities, including memory.

misindentification The perception that a familiar face, animal, or object is someone or something different that is actually the case.

MoCA (montreal cognitive assessment) It is a screening tool for mild cognitive dysfunction, including early onset of Alzheimer's. It assesses concentration, attention, memory, language, calculations, orientation, executive functions, and visual skills.

neuropsychological tests Mental tests (such as SLUMS) used to assess functions of the brain, such as language, problem solving, and memory.

rapid eye movement (REM) It is a sleep behavior disorder. A condition in which an individual experiences violent or frightening dreams and acts them out during sleep.

SLUMS The acronym stands for Saint Louis University Mental Status. It is designed to identify individuals with mild or early dementia through measuring orientation, memory, attention, and executive functions.

spatial disorientation Loss of an individual's sense of place that may cause difficulties knowing where one is while driving, while in a store, others buildings, or home.

virtual dementia tour It is an experience that allows participants to encounter many of the symptoms that people suffering from dementia undergo daily.

Resources

Google Specifics (not an exhaustive list)

AARP African American/Black Faith Based Initiative Tool
Kit
AARP Memory Activity Book
ACTS2 Tallahassee, Florida
Alzheimer's Association "The Brains Behind Yours"
American Association Retired People (AARP)
African Americans, Latinos, Veterans, Faith, and
Hispanics Us Against Alzheimer's
Alzheimer's Disease and related Dementias Education and
Referral Center (ADEAR) 1 800 438-4380
Alzheimer's Society
Alzstore.com
Bright Focus Foundation "Cure in Mind. Cure in Sight"
Caring Kind
Clinical Trials in your State
Dementia Action Alliance
Dementia & Alzheimer's Wellbeing Network (DAWN)
Dementia Friends
Dementia Matters
Dementia Spotlight Foundation
Dementia Today
Emory University

Fearless Caregiver
Glenner Town Square
Global Brain Health Institute
Healthline
Home Health Care Services
Hospice Services
In Our Right Mind (documentary by Renee Chenault-
    Fattah, JD)
Mayo Clinic
Memory Café
Memory Care Facilities
Military Families Ensure your attorney specializes in Elder
    Care Law and Veterans Special Pensions Aid and
    Assistance.
Nonmedical Home Care Services
Public Health Services
Respite Care or Adult Care Centers
Salud America!
Second Wind Dreams
Senior Companions
State Funded Care Giving Programs
Support Groups in your area (i.e., Dementia Support
    Groups, Alzheimer's Support Groups)
Teepa Snow
WebMD
Women's Alzheimer's Movement
YOUR personal family and friends

Informed Consent Form

Print Your Name
I, _________________________________ understand
the author **Debra Tann** is writing a book. I have agreed to
allow her to articulate on paper, my story.

I understand the tenants established by **Debra Tann**
and the conditions of my interview. Moreover, I have the
authority to edit the information contained therein to
ensure that it is factual and properly reflects my thoughts.
I further understand my identity will not be disclosed.

By signing this form, I give my consent as a
participant to share my story in her book.

Participant Signature _________________________________
Author (Debra Tann) Signature _________________________
Date _________________________________

References

Alzheimer's Association (2019). *Dementia Types.*
http://www.alz.org

Alzheimer's Association (2019). *Dementia Related.*
http://www.alz.org

Alzheimer's Association (2019). *Alzheimer's-Dementia
Facts and Figures.* http://www.alz.org

Alzheimer's Association. (2002). *African Americans and
Alzheimer's Disease: The Silent Epidemic*, 2002.
Retrieved from http://www.alz.org

Alzheimer's Association (2010, March 8). *New report says
African-Americans and Hispanics more likely to have
Alzheimer's disease than Whites.* http://www.alz.org

Alzheimer's Association (2019). *Women and Alzheimer's.*
http://alz.org

Alzheimer's Association AAIC Press Office. (2018).
*Pregnancy and Reproductive History May Impact
Dementia Risk Plus, the Move to Re-Think the Impact
of Hormone Therapy on Cognition* [Women and
dementia]. Retrieved from http://www.alz.org/aaic/
releases_2018

Alzheimer's Association. (2014). [*communication*].
Chicago, USA: Alzheimer's Association.

Alzheimer's Association. (2014). [*legal plans*].
Chicago, USA: Alzheimer's Association.

Alzheimer's Association. (2014). [*take care of yourself*]. Chicago, USA: Alzheimer's Association.

Alzheimer's Association. (2018). *Dementia and Driving.* http://alz.org

Alzheimer's Association. (2018). [10 Warning Signs of Alzheimer's Disease]. Chicago, USA: Alzheimer's Association.

Alzheimer's Association Press Office. (2018). *Congress Takes BOLD Steps in Fight to Address Alzheimer's* [Congressional presence]. Retrieved from http://www.alz.org/news

Alzheimer's Society (2016, May). *Genetics of dementia.* http://www.alzheimers.org

Alzheimer's Society (2017, August). *7 Things not to say to somebody with dementia.* http://alzheimers.org

American Association of Retired Persons (2018, June 25). *New Survey: Doctors Feel Defeated by Dementia.* https://www.aarp.org/health/dementia/info-2018

American Heart Association (2019, January 9). *AHA: Blood Pressure May Explain Higher Dementia Risk in Blacks.* https://consumer.healthday.com

Avramova, N., (2019). *Blood test could detect Alzheimer's up to 16 years before symptom begin, study says.* https://www.cnn.com/2019/01/22/

Clarity Pointe (2018). *7 Ways to Cope with a Parent's Diagnosis of Dementia.* http://www.claritypointe.com

Ellison, J. M., (2017). *The Burden of Alzheimer's Disease on African Americans.* http://www.brightfocus.org

Emory University (2016, November 9). *Spotlight: Alzheimer's and the African American Community.* https://healthyaging.emory.edu

Fritten LJ, Ortiz F, Ponton M. *Frequency of Alzheimer's disease and other dementias in a community outreach sample of Hispanics.* J Am Geriatr Soc 2001;49(10):1301-8.

Golden, M. (2019). *On B. Smith, Husband Dan Gasby and the Blacklash Over Moving On When a Spouse Has Alzheimer's.* http://www.theglowup.theroot.com

Heerema, E. (2017, May 27) *How was Alzheimer's Disease Discovered?* http://www.verywellhealth.com

Mayo Foundation for Medical Education and Research (1998-2019). *Dementia Symptoms and Causes.* http://www.mayoclinic.org

National Hispanic Council on Aging. (2013 & 2105). *Status of Hispanic Older Adults.* http://latinosaganistalzheimers.org

Richmond, M., (2007). [*Dealing with Anger*]. Santa Cruz, USA: Journey Works Publishing.

Salud America! (2019, April 18). *The CHANGE Act on Alzheimer's: How Will It Impact Latinos?* https://salud-america.org

Sauer, A., (2018, November 21). Study Identifies Biggest Alzheimer's Caregiver Challenges. Retrieved March 24, 2019, from https://www.alzheimers.net

Science Daily (2018, April 9). *Controlling blood pressure even when older can prevent dementia in African Americans.* https://www.sciencedaily.com

UsAganistAlzheimer's. (2019). *CURING ALZHEIMER'S CLINICAL TRIALS are the KEY*, 2019. Retrieved from http://www.UsAganistAlzheimers.org/research

UsAganistAlzheimer's Press Office. (2019). *UsAganistAlzheimer's Applauds the Bipartisan Introduction of the CHANGE Act, Critical Legislation to Promote Early Diagnosis of Alzheimer's* [Organization applauds bipartisanship]. Retrieved from https://www.usaganistalzheimers.org/press

UsAgainstAlzheimer's. (2019). *Latinos & Alzheimer's Disease: New Numbers Behind the Crisis*, 2019. Retrieved from http://www.UsAganistAlzheimers.org

About the Author

Dr. Debra Tann is originally from Sacramento, California. Dr. Tann and her husband moved to Valdosta (via military) twenty-five years ago when all three of their sons were under the age of five. Fast forward…their oldest son graduated from Yale University and is married to a Yale graduate and Rhodes scholar. Their middle son graduated from the University of North Georgia and is degreed in Criminal Justice. He is married to a middle grade's history teacher. Their youngest son graduated from Toccoa Falls Christian College and is in the business world. He is married to his college sweetheart who is degreed in the performing arts. Dr. Tann is married to a retired and career navy man. Currently, they travel and celebrate one granddaughter who happens to be 2 years old as of this writing.

Professionally, Dr. Tann has taught at the community college level as a political science educator. Thereafter, she went on to teach at the university level after obtaining her doctorate degree in Education Administration and Leadership. Dr. Tann's dissertation was entitled "The Effects of Developmental Education Programs for Service Members in the United State Military." Her dissertation produced groundbreaking research that subsequently garnered her opportunities to present at national conferences in the United States. Dr. Tann also has life-long credentials and certifications in Community College, Adult Basic Education, and Competency Based Education. Moreover, she is nationally certified in Differentiated Learning Styles and is recognized as Who's Who in the Southeast.

In 2002, Dr. Tann planned, implemented, and executed a private independent school called Genesis Christian School. Her middle son, who was in the third grade, questioned her colossal project by stating "no one starts a school." He was correct in that it was a special calling from the Lord. Genesis Christian School was groundbreaking in that it supported itself solitarily (no governmental financial assistance) throughout its tenure. This task commanded enormous competence, dedication, and faith. The school impacted many lives that sought to meet students at their Genesis. It also won "Small Business of the Year."

What is more, Genesis relocated from leasing a 5,500 square foot property to purchasing a forty thousand-square-foot campus nestled on nine acres of fenced property. The school boasted thirty-three classrooms, full gymnasium with wood floors, a 2,300 square footage library, a state-of-the-art kitchen/cafeteria, and much more.

Genesis' reputation remains a pillar in the community that set the standard of educational excellence uncompromised. She credits the Lord for His unwavering favor, her family for their unfaltering commitment, and her extended family and friends who believed and supported the vision of Genesis Christian School.

Dr. Tann is qualified in the areas of strategic planning, coalition building, program planning, organizational implementation, execution, and evaluation. She has experience with faculty and staff development, interpersonal skills, fundraising acumen, fiscal competence, listening, a sense of humor, visionary skills, and unrivaled administrative and organizational skills. Most recently and post Genesis, Dr. Tann has served as an educational consultant with a specialization as a strategist and coach. However, the last four years of her life has been and continues to be dedicated to advocating on behalf of families whose loved ones have dementia. Her passion resides in this area, and she seeks to make a difference through the education of brain health. As a person of color, Dr. Tann is desirous of educating minority families such as Blacks (African Americans), Hispanics, and Latinos who have unparalleled data concluding the dramatic increase of one of the dementias.

On the lighter side, Dr. Tann enjoys theatrical plays, stand-up comics, and traveling nationally and internationally. Dr. Tann enjoys watching C-Span, the Travel Station, NPR, To Tell the Truth, Judge Judy, and news stations on television. What is more, she loves God, her husband, sons/wives, granddaughter, and intellectual conversations. Musically speaking, her genres of music styles include jazz, old school music (particularly the Motown era), classical, and gospel music. During Dr. Tann's relaxing times, she prefers strolls along the seashore and reading. She likes island beaches, laughter, bright colors, games, and Chinese and Soul food.

Her favorite Christian writers are Tony Evans and Billy Graham. Her favorite thinkers include Cornell West, Martin Luther King Jr., Maya Angelou, W. E. B. Du Bois, Alain Locke, and Toni Morrison. Dr. Tann is also a "quote" enthusiast. She said they encourage her to think critically, and they are inspirational.

Dr. Tann has and continues to mentor young women in her path. Many times, she is moved emotionally by individuals who articulate the profound influence she has had in their professional and/or personal life. Individuals who have impacted and influenced Dr. Tann's life include: Jesus, Dorothy Height, Mary McCloud Bethune, Barbara Jordan, and Mary Lee Hardy.

Dr. Debra Tann's priorities in life include God, studying His Word, and her family. Her servanthood and zeal is to influence and impact the lives of others. Cicely Tyson once said, and Dr. Tann concurs, "If one benefits more than the people they serve; they are no longer servants."

Follow Dr. Debra Tann on her Podcast at DebraonDementia.com

Follow Dr. Debra Tann on Twitter at DebraonDementia and on Linkedin.com

For speaking engagements contact Dr. Tann at her email address: dr.debra.tann@gmail.com